PICKLING AND FERMENTING COOKBOOK

A Comprehensive Beginner's Friendly Handbook On Pickling And Fermenting With Mouthwatering Recipes For All Skill Levels.

By

ELLA R. SMITH

Copyright page

Pickling And Fermenting Cookbook:A Comprehensive Beginner's Friendly Handbook On Pickling And Fermenting With Mouthwatering Recipes For All Skill Levels.
Copyright © 2023 Ella R. Smith

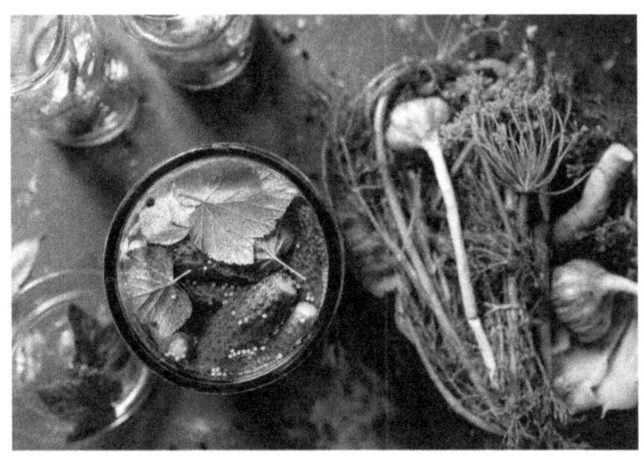

Introduction

Hi there! Welcome to our "Pickling and Fermenting Cookbook"! If you've ever been curious about turning everyday ingredients into something extraordinary, you're in for a treat.

This cookbook is all about pickling and fermenting—two age-old methods that make food not only taste fantastic but also boost its goodness. Don't worry if you're new to this; we're here to guide you through every step. And if you're already a kitchen pro, get ready for some exciting new recipes!

This cookbook explains every concept in the pickling and fermenting world that beginners need to familiarize themselves with.

Inside these pages, you'll find a mix of classic favorites and fresh ideas. From crunchy pickles to zesty fermented fruits, there's something for everyone. We've kept things simple, so you can dive right in, whether you're a beginner or a seasoned chef.

So, why pickling and fermenting? Well, besides making your taste buds dance, these techniques pack a nutritional punch. Probiotics, vitamins, and more—it's like a health boost for your kitchen creations!

Ready to join us on a flavor-filled adventure? Our cookbook is not just about recipes; it's an invitation to explore a world where jars hold treasures of deliciousness. Let's get pickling and fermenting; your tastebuds will thank you!

CHAPTER 1: INTRODUCTION TO PICKLING AND FERMENTATION

Welcome to the foundational chapter of our culinary journey, where we demystify the art of pickling and fermentation.

1.1 Understanding the Basics of Pickling and Fermentation!

Pickling

Imagine a fortress protecting your food, not with stone and steel but with a moat of zesty vinegar or a briny ocean of salt. That's pickling! This age-old method bathes food in an acidic solution, creating a formidable barrier against spoilage-causing bacteria.

Pickling, a culinary craft spanning centuries, is the art of preserving foods—vegetables and fruits—in an acidic solution, often vinegar, or a salt solution known as brine. The preserving magic, especially with salt, involves fermentation, where lactic acid plays a key role. Commonly known as brining, the delightful outcomes are universally referred to as pickles. In North America, "pickles" primarily conjure thoughts of cucumber pickles, but the method extends to eggs, meat, and fish, termed curing. The spectrum of pickled vegetables is vast, from olives to cabbage, cucumbers, cauliflower, carrots, beans, capers, onions, and garlic, each boasting unique flavors. In Asian countries, kimchi takes the stage as a tradition deeply rooted in Korea.

Fermentation:

What is fermentation?

While the mention of fermentation often invokes images of wine and beer production, the process extends far beyond the brewing realm. Lacto-fermentation, the transformative technique behind fermented foods like kimchi and kombucha, involves the conversion of sugars into lactic acid by lactobacillus bacteria. These beneficial bacteria not only preserve the food but also promote digestive health, offering a rich source of probiotics. The fermented foods resulting from this process become culinary allies, contributing to the well-being of our bodies.

Fermentation's Magical Toolkit:

Lactic Acid: The tangy alchemist, a product of the microbial feast, preserves and adds a signature pucker.

Probiotics are friendly bacteria warriors, strengthening your gut's defenses and fostering digestive harmony.

Starter Cultures: A boost for the alchemists, these concentrated packs of good bacteria jumpstart the fermentation process.

1.2 Difference between pickling and fermenting

Pickling and fermentation share commonalities, yet they represent distinct methods of food preservation. Both processes involve the use of a brine solution, typically consisting of water and salt, to create an environment conducive to microbial activity. In pickling, the acidity usually comes from the addition of vinegar, creating a tangy flavor profile. On the other hand, fermentation relies on the natural production of acids, often lactic acid, by beneficial microorganisms like lactobacillus. While both techniques use salt to inhibit the growth of harmful bacteria, fermentation takes advantage of the naturally occurring microbes to initiate the process. Essentially, fermentation is a broader category that encompasses pickling, as vegetables and fruits that undergo pickling often go through a fermentation process facilitated by these microorganisms. So, while pickling involves brining for preservation, fermentation is the overarching biological transformation that certain pickled foods undergo, where the microbes play a pivotal role in enhancing flavors and nutritional content.

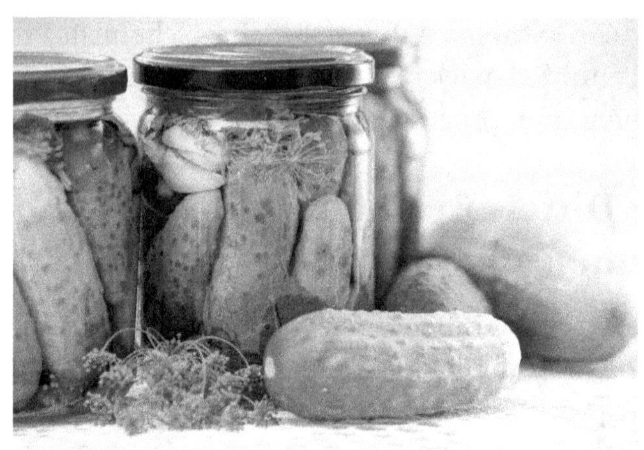

CHAPTER 2: GETTING STARTED

This invites you into the heart of culinary exploration, unraveling the basics for a delightful journey into the art of pickling and fermenting."

2.1 Quick Pickling vs. Traditional Pickling

In the realm of pickling, two distinct techniques offer unique advantages and flavors. Let's explore the differences between quick pickling and traditional pickling, each bringing its own charm to the world of preserved delights.

1. Quick Pickling:

Quick pickling, also known as refrigerator pickling or fresh pickling, is the swift counterpart to its traditional counterpart. As the name suggests, this method skips the lengthy fermentation process, allowing you to enjoy tangy pickles in a matter of hours.

Process:

Vegetables are sliced or chopped.

A simple brine, often consisting of vinegar, water and salt heated and poured over the vegetables.

The jars are then refrigerated for a relatively short period, typically a few hours to overnight.

Advantages:

Quick results: Perfect for those craving pickles without the wait.

Retains crispness: Vegetables maintain a crunchy texture due to the brief brining period.

Versatility: Experiment with various flavors and spice combinations easily.

Popular Quick Pickle Choices:

Red onions with balsamic vinegar and herbs.

Radishes with rice vinegar and sesame seeds.

Cucumbers with dill and white vinegar.

2. Traditional Pickling:

Traditional pickling, often associated with fermentation, is a slower but transformative process. It involves the natural fermentation of vegetables in a brine over an extended period, resulting in complex flavors and the introduction of beneficial bacteria.

Process:

Vegetables are prepared and packed into jars.

A brine, typically consisting of water, salt, and sometimes additional flavorings, is poured over the vegetables.

The jars are left at room temperature for an extended period, ranging from several days to weeks, allowing fermentation to occur.

Advantages:

Depth of flavor: Fermentation introduces complex and tangy flavors.

Probiotic benefits: The presence of beneficial bacteria supports digestive health.

Longer shelf life: Traditional pickles can be stored for an extended period of time.

Popular Traditional Pickle Choices:

Classic dill pickles with garlic and spices.

Sauerkraut, fermented cabbage, and caraway seeds.

Kimchi, a spicy Korean staple with Napa cabbage and chili.

Two other types of pickling methods are:

1.Vinegar brine method

The vinegar brine method in pickling is a preservation technique where food items are immersed in a solution of vinegar, water, salt, and often sugar, along with various herbs and spices. The acidity of the vinegar acts as a natural preservative, preventing the growth of spoilage microorganisms. The brine imparts a tangy and flavorful taste to the pickled items. This method is commonly used for pickling vegetables, such as cucumbers, and involves preparing the brine, packing the vegetables into sterilized jars, and pouring the brine over them. The sealed jars can be stored in a cool, dark place, allowing the flavors to develop over time.

2. Water Bath Method

The water bath method of pickling is a canning technique used to preserve high-acid foods, such as pickles and fruits, in glass jars. It involves immersing filled jars in a boiling water bath for a specific period of time. This process creates a vacuum seal, preventing the growth of spoilage microorganisms and ensuring the long-term shelf stability of the pickled items. The sealed jars can be stored in a cool, dark place until they are ready for use.

2.2 Key Ingredients for Pickling

Embarking on a journey into the world of pickling and fermentation requires a careful selection of ingredients. Whether you're aiming for crisp pickles or tangy sauerkraut, these key ingredients form the building blocks of your culinary adventure:

1. Vegetables and Fruits:

Cucumbers: A classic choice for pickling, cucumbers transform into delightful pickles.

Cabbage: Essential for sauerkraut, cabbage undergoes a flavorful fermentation process.

Carrots, Radishes, and More: Diverse vegetables lend their unique textures and flavors to the mix.

Fruits: Apples, pears, and even berries can be pickled or fermented for a sweet twist.

2. Salt:

Sea Salt or Kosher Salt: Unrefined salts work well for pickling and fermentation, providing essential minerals.

3. Vinegar:

White vinegar is a versatile option for pickling vegetables, offering a sharp tang.

Apple Cider Vinegar: It adds a nuanced flavor and is commonly used in various pickling recipes.

4. Spices and herbs:

Dill is a classic herb for pickles, lending a fresh and aromatic note.

Mustard Seeds: Add a distinctive flavor profile to pickled vegetables.

Garlic infused depth and savory undertones.

Coriander Seeds, Peppercorns, and More: A medley of spices enriches the flavor palette.

5. Water:

Filtered water is essential for creating brine solutions and ensuring a clean environment for fermentation.

6. Optional enhancements:

Ginger adds warmth and complexity to both pickles and fermented foods.

Turmeric imparts a golden hue and earthy notes.

Chilies: Infuse heat for those who prefer a spicy kick.

Herbs like thyme or rosemary elevate the aromatic profile.

Remember, the beauty of pickling and fermentation lies in experimentation. Feel free to tweak these ingredients, explore new flavors, and make the process uniquely yours.

2.3 Essential Equipment for Pickling and their uses

1.   Glass Jars with Lids:

Use: To pack and store pickles.

2.   Weights or Fermentation Stones:

Use: Keep vegetables submerged during fermentation.

3. Airlocks:

Use: Allow gasses to escape without letting air in, maintaining an ideal pickling environment.

4. Brining Container with Airtight Lid:

Use: Mix and store brines efficiently.

5. Wooden Spoons or Tampers:

Use: Pack vegetables into jars and tamp down to remove air pockets.

6. Cheesecloth or coffee filters:

Use: Cover jars during fermentation, allowing gasses to escape while preventing contaminants.

7. pH Strips:

Use: Monitor acidity levels during fermentation for safety and flavor.

8. Cutting boards and knives:

Use: Prepare vegetables and fruits for pickling.

9. Non-Iodized Salt:

Use: Essential for creating brines without additives that could affect pickling.

10. Measuring Tools:

Use: accurate measurement of ingredients for consistent and safe pickling.

11. Labels and markers:

Use: Organize jars by labeling them with date, type, and any additional notes.

12. Clean towels or clothes:

Use: Cover jars during fermentation to protect them from light and debris.

Having these tools ensures a smooth and successful pickling process, from preparation to fermentation and storage.

2.4 Step by Step Guide to Pickling

Pickling Fruits and Vegetables:

Pickling is a delightful journey of transforming ordinary fruits and vegetables into tangy, flavorful delights. Follow these step-by-step instructions for a foolproof pickling experience, complete with accurate measurements:

Ingredients:

Fresh fruits or vegetables (e.g., cucumbers, carrots, radishes, strawberries)

Non-iodized salt

White vinegar

Water

Sugar

Pickling spices (optional)

Fresh herbs (e.g., dill, garlic, mustard seeds) for flavor enhancement

Equipment:

Glass jars with wide mouths and lids

Weights or fermentation stones

Airlocks (optional but recommended)

Brining container with an airtight lid

Wooden spoons or tamper

Cheesecloth or coffee filters

pH strips

Cutting boards and knives

Measuring spoons and kitchen scale

Labels and waterproof markers

Clean towels or cloth

Step 1: Prepare Your Ingredients

Choose fresh produce:

Select fresh, crisp fruits or vegetables. Rinse them thoroughly, and trim or slice as desired.

Step 2: Sterilize Your Equipment

Clean Jars and Lids:

Start cleaning jars and lid by using hot soapy water to wash them thoroughly and properly then rinse thoroughly too. Sterilize by boiling rubber seals and metal lids for ten minutes. Allow them to air-dry.

Step 3: Create a Brine Solution

Calculate the brine ratio:

For a basic brine, use 1 tablespoon of non-iodized salt per quart of water. Adjust based on your taste preferences.

Step 4: Pack Your Jars

Layer Fruits or Vegetables:

Pack your jars with the prepared fruits or vegetables. Add any desired fresh herbs, pickling spices, or aromatics.

Step 5: Pour in the brine

Fill Jars with Brine:

Pour the prepared brine over the fruits or vegetables, ensuring they are fully submerged. Leave approximately 1 inch of headspace.

Step 6: Weigh down and cover

Add Weights or Fermentation Stones:

Place weights or fermentation stones to keep the fruits or vegetables submerged. Cover the jars with lids and, if using, airlocks.

Step 7: Monitor Fermentation

Set the stage for fermentation:

Place the jars in a cool, dark place with a temperature between 65°F and 75°F (18°C to 24°C). Monitor the pH using strips and taste the pickles periodically.

Step 8: Label and Date Jars

Organize Your Pickle Pantry:

Label each jar with the date, type of pickle, and any additional notes. This helps you track aging and discover your favorite recipes.

Step 9: Taste and Adjust

Fine-Tune Flavors:

Taste your pickles as they ferment. Adjust salt, sweetness, or additional flavors as needed, using small amounts at a time.

Step 10: Store Properly

Preserve Your Pickles:

Once you are satisfied with the flavor, store the pickled items in clean, airtight jars in a cool, dark place. keep in the Refrigerator after opening for an extended shelf life.

Note: This step-by-step pickling guide for vegetables using a brine solution can be adapted for pickling with vinegar. Both methods essentially involve creating a preserving liquid to impart flavor and extend the shelf life of vegetables. The key difference is the acid used in the solution.

Here's a step-by-step explanation of the water bath method:

Prepare Jars and Lids:

Wash glass jars, lids, and bands in hot, soapy water. Rinse thoroughly.

Inspect Jars:

Check the jars for any cracks or chips. Discard any damaged jars to ensure a proper seal.

Sterilize Jars:

Place the jars in a boiling water bath or use a dishwasher to sterilize them. Jars should be Kept hot until ready for use.

Prepare the pickling recipe:

Follow your chosen pickling recipe, prepare the brine or vinegar solution, and pack the fruits or vegetables into the hot, sterilized jars.

Leave Headspace:

Ensure you leave the recommended headspace at the top of each jar, as specified in your recipe. This space allows for the expansion of contents during processing.

Wipe Jar Rims:

Before placing the lids on the jars, wipe the rims with a clean, damp cloth to remove any residue that could interfere with the seal.

Apply Lids and Bands:

Place the clean, sterilized lids on the jars and screw on the metal bands until they are fingertip-tight. Avoid over-tightening.

Prepare a water-bath canner.

Fill a water bath canner with enough water to cover the jars by at least 1 to 2 inches. Heat the water to a simmer, but not boiling.

Process Jars:

Carefully lower the filled jars into the simmering water bath using a jar lifter. Ensure the jars are fully submerged.

Process for Recommended Time:

Process the jars for the recommended time specified in your pickling recipe. The processing time may vary based on the type of food and the size of the jar.

Remove Jars:

Once the processing time is complete, use the jar lifter to remove the jars from the water bath canner and place them on a clean, dry towel or cooling rack.

Cooling and sealing:

Allow the jars to cool undisturbed. As they cool, the lids should make a popping sound, indicating a proper seal. Check for a concave indentation in the lid, indicating a vacuum seal.

Check Seals:

Once cooled, apply pressure to the middle of each lid. If it doesn't pop back and you can't press it down further, the jar is properly sealed. If a lid flexes, refrigerate the jar and consume its contents promptly.

Label and Store:

Label the sealed jars with the date and type of pickled food. Keep the jars in a cool, dark place.

The water bath method is effective for preserving high-acid foods, creating a safe and shelf-stable environment for your pickled creations.

2.5 Troubleshooting and FAQs on Pickling

1. Why are my pickles too soft?

Issue: overripe or soft vegetables, insufficient salt, or improper water-to-vinegar ratio.

Solution: Use fresh, crisp vegetables, ensure proper salt concentration, and maintain the recommended brine ratio.

2. Why is the brine cloudy?

Issue: iodized salt, minerals in water, or insufficiently dissolved salt.

Solution: Use non-iodized salt, use filtered water, and ensure the salt is fully dissolved.

3. What causes mold on the surface?

Issue: exposure to air, contaminated equipment, or insufficient brine coverage.

Solution: Ensure vegetables are fully submerged, use weights or fermentation stones, and maintain a clean environment.

4. Why are my pickles too salty?

Issue: overuse of salt or not rinsing salted vegetables before pickling.

Solution: Follow the recommended salt ratios and rinse salted vegetables thoroughly.

5. Why are my pickles not tangy enough?

Issue: insufficient fermentation time or low acidity in the brine.

Solution: Allow more time for fermentation or increase the vinegar content in the brine.

6. What causes spongy pickles?

Issue: improper cucumber selection, overripe cucumbers, or inconsistent sizing.

Solution: Choose firm cucumbers, ensure uniform sizing, and pick at the right stage of ripeness.

7. Why did my lids not seal properly?

Issue: Jar rims not cleaned properly, over-tightened bands, or old lids.

Solution: Clean jar rims thoroughly, avoid over-tightening bands, and use new, undamaged lids.

8. Can I reuse pickling brine?

Answer: It's not recommended for water bath canning due to potential changes in acidity. For refrigerator pickles, reuse cautiously, but fresh brine is preferable for canning.

9. How long do pickled vegetables last?

Answer: Properly sealed and stored pickled vegetables can last for up to a year or more. Check if there are signs of spoilage before consuming.

10. Can I adjust the spices in my pickling recipe?

Answer: Yes, feel free to experiment with spices, but avoid altering the vinegar-to-water ratio as it affects acidity and preservation.

2.6 Navigating Fermentation Techniques

As we delve deeper into the art of food fermentation, it becomes essential to understand the diverse methods that shape the alchemy of transformation. Each technique brings its own unique nuances, giving rise to a spectrum of flavors and textures that define the culinary wonders of fermentation.

Lacto-Fermentation:

Lacto Fermentation takes center stage, a process where lactobacillus bacteria convert sugars into lactic acid. This method is renowned for its ability to both preserve and enhance flavors, as seen in classics like sauerkraut and kimchi. The tangy outcome is not only a treat for the taste buds but also a source of probiotics, contributing to digestive well-being.

Yeast-Fermentation:

In the world of fermentation, yeast-driven alchemy transforms sugars into alcohol and carbon dioxide. This method extends beyond the realms of brewing, playing a pivotal role in the creation of bread. The rise and texture of a perfectly baked loaf owe their magic to the transformative power of yeast.

Acetic acid fermentation:

Acetic acid fermentation, the force behind vinegar, adds a distinct tanginess to the culinary repertoire. Acetobacter bacteria convert ethanol into acetic acid, shaping the character of both vinegar and foods like kombucha. The effervescence of this process contributes not only to taste but also to the refreshing qualities of fermented beverages.

Wild Fermentation:

Venturing into the spontaneity of wild fermentation, the natural microorganisms present in the environment take the lead. This unscripted method yields unique and complex flavors, elevating foods like naturally fermented sourdough bread and artisanal cheeses to new heights. Here, the terroir of microorganisms becomes an integral part of the culinary narrative.

Understanding these fermentation techniques reveals the artistry behind the culinary craft. From the controlled dance of lacto-fermentation to the untamed elegance of wild fermentation, each method presents an opportunity for creativity and exploration. As we navigate this intricate tapestry of techniques, the rich world of fermented foods unfolds, inviting us to savor the myriad possibilities within each transformative process.

Note: Many of the essential pieces of equipment for fermentation are also commonly used in pickling. The crossover between pickling and fermentation equipment is because both processes share similar principles and requirements.

CHAPTER 3: HEALTH BENEFITS OF PICKLED AND FERMENTED FOODS

In understanding the health aspects of pickled and fermented foods, it's crucial to recognize their nutritional value. The process of fermentation, driven by beneficial microorganisms, not only enhances the flavors but also preserves essential nutrients. This preservation often results in increased concentrations of vitamins and minerals.

Exploring the Nutritional Value of Fermented Foods

A key nutritional aspect of fermented foods is the presence of probiotics. These live microorganisms, cultivated during fermentation, play a significant role in supporting gut health. By colonizing the digestive tract, they contribute to maintaining a balanced microbiome, aiding in digestion and nutrient absorption.

Fermented foods can also be rich in B vitamins, which are crucial for energy metabolism and overall well-being. Additionally, the fermentation process may break down anti-nutrients present in certain foods, making nutrients more accessible.

Sauerkraut, kimchi, pickles, and other fermented foods aren't just flavorful additions to our meals;

they serve as functional foods, offering taste along with potential health benefits. Examining the nutritional value of fermented foods reveals their role in supporting our well-being, providing more reasons to enjoy these foods beyond their taste.

Gut Health and Fermentation

Delving into the intricate relationship between gut health and fermentation reveals a fascinating interplay that significantly impacts overall well-being. The gut, often referred to as the "second brain," plays a pivotal role in our immune system, nutrient absorption, and even mental health.

The Gut Microbiome: A Microscopic Ecosystem

At the heart of this connection is the gut microbiome—an intricate ecosystem teeming with trillions of microorganisms, including bacteria, fungi, and viruses. Fermented foods contribute to this ecosystem by introducing probiotics, beneficial bacteria that exert positive effects on gut health.

Probiotics: Nurturing Microbial Harmony

The probiotics derived from fermented foods act as reinforcements for the gut's microbial army. They help maintain a balance between good and potentially harmful bacteria, creating an environment conducive to optimal digestion and nutrient absorption. This microbial harmony doesn't just impact the gut; it resonates throughout the body, influencing various aspects of health.

Fermented Foods as Gut Supporters

Sauerkraut, yogurt, kefir, and other fermented delights act as allies in nurturing a thriving gut environment. The lactic acid bacteria produced during fermentation work in tandem with the existing gut flora, promoting diversity and resilience. As these beneficial microorganisms flourish, they contribute to the synthesis of essential nutrients and the breakdown of certain compounds, which might be challenging for the digestive system.

Beyond Digestion: Fermentation and Immune Support

The impact of a healthy gut extends beyond digestion. The gut is a key player in our immune system, and the balance maintained by probiotics from fermented foods contributes to immune resilience. A well-supported gut is better equipped to defend against pathogens, potentially reducing the risk of infection and supporting overall immune function.

In unraveling the connection between gut health and fermentation, we uncover a realm where the foods we consume play a crucial role in fostering a resilient and thriving internal environment. As we explore the tangible benefits of incorporating fermented foods into our diets, the intricate dance between our gut and the microbial allies within becomes clearer, offering a path to enhanced well-being.

Other Health Benefits of Pickled and Fermented Foods

In addition to their impact on nutritional content, pickled and fermented foods offer various health advantages that haven't been previously highlighted:

Microbial Diversity: Fermented foods contribute to the diversity of the gut microbiome, supporting a broader range of beneficial microorganisms.

Reduced Anti-Nutrient Content: Fermentation can reduce the levels of anti-nutrients, compounds that may interfere with nutrient absorption in the digestive system.

Potential Antioxidant Formation: Some fermented foods may undergo processes that enhance the formation of antioxidants, which can help combat oxidative stress in the body.

Bioactive Compounds: Fermentation can generate bioactive compounds, such as peptides and organic acids, with potential health-promoting properties.

Improved Lactose Digestion: Fermented dairy products, like yogurt, may be better tolerated by individuals with lactose intolerance due to the action of probiotics on lactose.

Regulation of Appetite: Fermented foods may influence appetite regulation through their impact on gut hormones, potentially aiding in weight management.

Potential Anti-Inflammatory Effects: Some studies suggest that fermented foods may possess anti-inflammatory properties, contributing to overall inflammatory balance in the body.

These additional health benefits further underscore the multifaceted advantages of incorporating pickled and fermented foods into one's diet for a holistic approach to well-being.

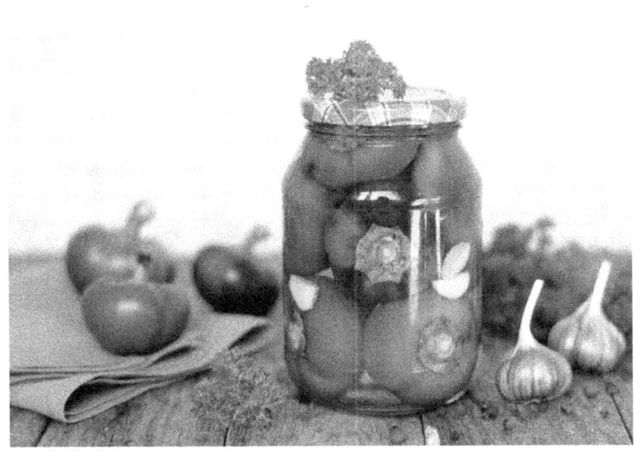

CHAPTER 4: PICKLED VEGETABLE RECIPES

Classic Dill Pickles

Description: Dive into the timeless appeal of classic dill pickles. Crisp and flavorful, these pickles are the perfect accompaniment to sandwiches, burgers, or enjoyed on their own as a satisfying snack.

Preparation Time: 15 minutes

Cook Time: 10 minutes

Servings: 8

Ingredients:

4 cups pickling cucumbers, sliced into spears or rounds

4 cloves of garlic, peeled and sliced

2 tablespoons of dill seeds

1 tablespoon of whole black peppercorns

2 cups of white vinegar

2 cups of water

3 tablespoons pickling salt

Fresh dill (optional)

Red pepper flakes (optional, for added heat)

Instructions:

Prepare Cucumbers:

Wash and slice the pickling cucumbers into desired shapes, such as spears or rounds.

Pack the jars:

Pack the sliced cucumbers into sterilized jars, leaving some space at the top.

Add Flavorings:

Distribute garlic slices, dill seeds, black peppercorns, and fresh dill (if using) evenly among the jars. Add a dash of pepper flakes for a hint of heat.

Prepare pickling liquid:

In a saucepan, combine white vinegar, water, and pickling salt. Bring everything in the pan to a boil over medium heat, ensuring the salt dissolves.

Pour hot pickling liquid:

Pour the hot pickling liquid into the jars, covering the cucumbers and flavors. Leave about 1/2 inch of headspace.

Seal the Jars:

Use a clean, damp cloth to wipe the jar rims and rim areas. Cover the jars with the sterilized lids, and screw on the bands until fingertip-tight.

Process for Canning (Optional):

If canning, process the jars in a hot water bath for 10 minutes to ensure a secure seal.

Storage:

Allow the classic dill pickles cool to room temperature.

Store the jars in a cool, dark place for at least 2 weeks for optimal flavor development.

Alternatively, refrigerate for at least 24 hours for a quicker infusion.

Tips for beginners:

Choose Fresh Cucumbers: Opt for firm and fresh pickling cucumbers for crisp pickles.

Sterilize Properly: Ensure jars, lids, and utensils are properly sterilized for a safe pickling process.

Experiment with Heat: Customize the level of heat by adjusting the amount of red pepper flakes.

Health Benefits:

Low-Calorie Snack: Dill pickles are a low-calorie snack option.

Hydration from Cucumbers: Cucumbers contribute to hydration due to their high water content.

Probiotic Potential: While these pickles are not fermented, they still offer a crunchy and flavorful addition to your diet.

Bread and butter pickles

Description: Experience the sweet and tangy delight of these classic bread and butter pickles. A perfect companion to sandwiches, burgers, or as a delightful side, these pickles add a touch of nostalgia to your culinary creations.

Preparation Time: 15 minutes

Cook Time: 10 minutes

Servings: 8

Ingredients:

4 cups thinly sliced cucumbers

1 large onion, thinly sliced

1/4 cup pickling salt

1 1/2 cups white vinegar

1 cup granulated sugar

1 tablespoon of mustard seeds

1 teaspoon of celery seeds

1/2 teaspoon turmeric

Ice cubes

Instructions:

Prepare the cucumbers and onions.

Thinly slice cucumbers and onions. Place them in a large bowl and sprinkle with pickling salt. Cover with ice cubes and let sit for 1-2 hours. Rinse and drain thoroughly.

Prepare pickling liquid:

In a saucepan, combine white vinegar, granulated sugar, mustard seeds, celery seeds, and turmeric. Bring everything in the pan to a boil over medium heat, stirring until the sugar dissolves.

Pack the jars:

Pack the sliced cucumbers and onions into sterilized jars.

Pour hot pickling liquid:

Pour the pickling liquid over the cucumbers and onions, ensuring they are fully submerged. Leave about 1/2 inch of headspace.

Seal the Jars:

Use a clean, damp cloth to wipe the rims and rim areas of the jars. Cover the jars with the sterilized lids, and screw on the bands until fingertip-tight.

Process for Canning (Optional):

If you're canning, process the jars in a hot water bath for 10 minutes for a secure seal.

Storage:

Allow the bread and butter pickles to cool to room temperature.

Store the jars in a cool, dark place for at least 2 weeks for optimal flavor development.

Alternatively, refrigerate for at least 24 hours for a quicker infusion.

Tips for beginners:

Use Fresh Cucumbers: Opt for fresh, firm cucumbers for the best texture in your pickles.

Follow Sterilization Guidelines: Properly sterilize jars, lids, and utensils for safe pickling.

Rinse Thoroughly: Ensure thorough rinsing of cucumbers and onions after the salting process to remove excess salt.

Health Benefits:

Cucumber Hydration: Cucumbers are hydrating and contain essential vitamins.

Moderation with Sugar: While sugar is used for flavor, it's essential to consume pickles in moderation for a balanced diet.

Classic Flavor Profile: Bread and butter pickles offer a classic, sweet-and-tangy flavor that appeals to various taste preferences.

Versatile Pairing: These pickles complement a wide range of dishes, making them a versatile addition to your kitchen.

Spicy Pickled Carrots

Description: Heat up your palate with these spicy pickled carrots. A fiery addition to tacos, sandwiches, or a standalone snack, these pickled carrots bring a bold and zesty kick to your culinary repertoire.

Preparation Time: 15 minutes

Cook Time: 10 minutes

Servings: 8

Ingredients:

1 pound of fresh carrots, peeled and sliced into sticks

2 cups of white vinegar

1 cup of water

2 tablespoons pickling salt

1 tablespoon of sugar

2 cloves of garlic, peeled and sliced

1 teaspoon crushed red pepper flakes

1 teaspoon whole black peppercorns

2 sprigs of fresh cilantro

Instructions:

Prepare Carrots:

Peel and slice carrots into sticks, ensuring they fit comfortably into your sterilized jars.

Prepare Brine:

In a saucepan, combine white vinegar, water, pickling salt, sugar, garlic, crushed red pepper flakes, and black peppercorns.

Bring everything in the pan to a boil over medium heat, stirring until the sugar and salt dissolve.

Pack the jars:

Pack the carrot sticks into sterilized jars, adding a sprig of fresh cilantro to each jar.

Pour hot brine:

Pour the hot brine over the carrot sticks, ensuring they are fully submerged. Leave about 1/2 inch of headspace.

Seal the Jars:

Use a clean, damp cloth to wipe the rims and rim areas of the jars with a clean, damp cloth. Cover the jars with the sterilized lids, and screw on the bands until fingertip-tight.

Process for Canning (Optional):

If you're canning, process the jars in a hot water bath for 10 minutes to ensure a proper seal.

Storage:

Allow the spicy pickled carrots to cool to room temperature.

Store the jars in a cool, dark place for at least 2 weeks for optimal flavor development.

Alternatively, refrigerate for at least 24 hours for a quicker infusion.

Tips for beginners:

Choose Fresh Carrots: Opt for fresh and crisp carrots for the best texture in your pickles.

Follow Sterilization Guidelines: Properly sterilize jars, lids, and utensils to ensure a safe pickling process.

Adjust Spice Level: Experiment with the amount of crushed red pepper flakes based on your spice preference. Start with a smaller amount for milder pickles.

Health Benefits:

Carrot Nutrients: Carrots are rich in beta-carotene, vitamins, and fiber.

Garlic's Potential Health Benefits: Garlic may contribute to cardiovascular health and provide immune system support.

Spice for Flavor and Metabolism: Crushed red pepper flakes not only add heat but may boost metabolism and provide anti-inflammatory benefits.

Cilantro Freshness: Cilantro not only enhances flavor but may also offer antioxidants and aid in digestion.

Sweet and Tangy Pickled Beets

Description: Indulge in the sweet and tangy symphony of these pickled beets. Perfect as a standalone snack, a colorful addition to salads, or paired with creamy goat cheese on a charcuterie board.

Preparation Time: 20 minutes

Cook Time: 30 minutes

Servings: 8

Ingredients:

3 cups sliced beets, cooked and peeled

2 cups apple cider vinegar

1 cup of water

1 cup granulated sugar

1 tablespoon pickling salt

1 teaspoon whole cloves

1 teaspoon whole allspice

1 cinnamon stick

1 orange, thinly sliced

Instructions:

Prepare Beets:

Cook beets until tender, peel, and slice into desired shapes.

Prepare pickling liquid:

In a saucepan, combine apple cider vinegar, water, sugar, pickling salt, whole cloves, whole allspice, and a cinnamon stick.

Bring everything in the pan to a boil over medium heat, stirring until the sugar and salt dissolve.

Add orange slices.

Add thinly sliced orange to the pickling liquid, bringing a citrusy brightness to the beets.

Pack the jars:

Pack the sliced beets into sterilized jars, ensuring they are evenly distributed.

Pour hot pickling liquid:

Pour the already prepared pickling liquid over the beets, ensuring they are fully submerged. Leave about 1/2 inch of headspace.

Seal the Jars:

Use a clean, damp cloth to wipe the rims and rim areas of the jars. Cover the jars with the sterilized lids, and screw on the bands until fingertip-tight.

Process for Canning (Optional):

If you're canning, process the jars in a hot water bath for 10 minutes for a secure seal.

Storage:

Allow the sweet and tangy pickled beets to cool to room temperature.

Store the jars in a cool, dark place for at least 2 weeks for optimal flavor development.

Alternatively, refrigerate for at least 24 hours for a quicker infusion.

Tips for beginners:

Use Cooked Beets: Start with pre-cooked and peeled beets for convenience.

Follow Sterilization Guidelines: Ensure jars, lids, and utensils are properly sterilized for safe pickling.

Experiment with Citrus: The addition of orange slices brings a refreshing twist to the classic pickled beets.

Health Benefits:

Beet Nutrients: Beets are rich in essential nutrients like folate, manganese, and fiber.

Apple Cider Vinegar Benefits: Apple cider vinegar may have various health benefits, including aiding digestion and supporting blood sugar control.

Spices for Flavor and Health: Cloves, allspice, and cinnamon not only enhance flavor but may offer antioxidants and anti-inflammatory properties.

Vibrant and Versatile: Sweet and tangy pickled beets add a burst of color and flavor to a range of culinary creations.

Balsamic-Pickled Asparagus

Description: Elevate your asparagus experience with the rich and tangy notes of balsamic pickling. These pickled asparagus spears bring a sophisticated touch to salads, antipasto platters, or as a unique side dish.

Preparation Time: 15 minutes

Cook Time: 10 minutes

Servings: 8

Ingredients:

1 bunch of fresh asparagus, tough ends trimmed

2 cups balsamic vinegar

1 cup of water

2 tablespoons pickling salt

1 tablespoon of sugar

4 cloves of garlic, peeled and sliced

1 teaspoon of black peppercorns

1 teaspoon dried thyme

Instructions:

Prepare Asparagus:

Trim the tough ends of the asparagus to fit the height of your sterilized jars.

Prepare Balsamic Brine:

In a saucepan, combine balsamic vinegar, water, pickling salt, sugar, garlic, black peppercorns, and dried thyme.

Bring everything in the pan to a boil over medium heat, stirring until the sugar and salt dissolve.

Blanch Asparagus:

Blanch the trimmed asparagus in boiling water for 2 minutes. Drain and set aside.

Pack the jars:

Pack the blanched asparagus spears into sterilized jars.

Pour hot balsamic brine:

Pour the hot balsamic brine over the asparagus, ensuring they are fully submerged. Leave about 1/2 inch of headspace.

Seal the Jars:

Use a clean damp cloth to wipe the rims and rim areas of the jars. Cover the jars with the sterilized and screw on the bands until fingertip-tight.

Process for Canning (Optional):

If you're canning, process the jars in a hot water bath for 10 minutes to ensure a proper seal.

Storage:

Allow the pickled asparagus to cool to room temperature.

Store the jars in a cool, dark place for at least 2 weeks for optimal flavor development.

Alternatively, refrigerate for at least 24 hours for a quicker infusion.

Tips for beginners:

Use Fresh Asparagus: Opt for fresh and vibrant asparagus for the best pickling results.

Follow Sterilization Guidelines: Properly sterilize jars, lids, and utensils to ensure a safe pickling process.

Experiment with Herbs: Balsamic pickling provides a canvas for experimenting with herbs; try adding rosemary or tarragon for different flavor profiles.

Health Benefits:

Asparagus Nutrients: Asparagus is a low-calorie vegetable rich in vitamins A, C, and K, as well as folate.

Balsamic Vinegar Antioxidants: Balsamic vinegar may contribute antioxidants that support overall health.

Garlic's Potential Health Benefits: Garlic, a common pickling ingredient, may have cardiovascular and immune system benefits.

Versatile Culinary Addition: Balsamic-pickled asparagus offers a versatile and sophisticated culinary touch to various dishes..

Turmeric Cauliflower Pickles

Description: Embrace the golden hues of turmeric with these flavorful cauliflower pickles. Infused with aromatic spices, these pickles add a zesty kick to salads, grain bowls, or serve as a vibrant side dish.

Preparation Time: 20 minutes

Cook Time: 10 minutes

Servings: 8

Ingredients:

1 medium cauliflower, separated into florets

2 cups of white vinegar

1 cup of water

1/4 cup granulated sugar

2 tablespoons pickling salt

1 tablespoon ground turmeric

1 teaspoon of mustard seeds

1 teaspoon of cumin seeds

1/2 teaspoon coriander seeds

4 cloves of garlic, peeled and crushed

Instructions:

Prepare Cauliflower:

Separate the cauliflower into bite-sized florets.

Prepare Brine:

In a saucepan, combine white vinegar, water, sugar, pickling salt, ground turmeric, mustard seeds, cumin seeds, coriander seeds, and crushed garlic.

Bring everything in the pan to a boil, stirring until the sugar and salt dissolve.

Blanch Cauliflower:

Blanch the cauliflower florets in boiling water for 2 minutes. Drain and set aside.

Infuse Cauliflower:

Add the blanched cauliflower to the boiling brine. Simmer for about 5 minutes until the cauliflower is slightly tender but still has a crunch.

Pack the jars:

Pack the cauliflower into sterilized jars.

Pour hot brine:

Pour the hot turmeric-infused brine over the cauliflower, leaving about 1/2 inch of headspace.

Seal the Jars:

Wipe the rims of the jars, place sterilized lids, and screw on the bands until fingertip-tight.

Process for Canning (Optional):

If canning, process the jars in a hot water bath for 10 minutes to ensure proper sealing.

Storage:

Allow the pickled cauliflower to rest for at least 2 weeks in a cool, dark place for optimal flavor development.

Alternatively, refrigerate for at least 24 hours for a quicker infusion.

Tips for beginners:

Use Fresh Cauliflower: Opt for fresh cauliflower for the best texture.

Follow Sterilization Guidelines: Properly sterilize jars, lids, and utensils for a safe pickling process.

Balance Spices: Adjust the spice level to your preference; start with a smaller amount for milder pickles.

Health Benefits:

Cruciferous Goodness: Cauliflower is a cruciferous vegetable, rich in vitamins and fiber.

Anti-Inflammatory Turmeric: Turmeric is renowned for its anti-inflammatory properties and potential overall well-being contributions.

Spice Blend Digestion: The spice blend, including mustard seeds, cumin seeds, and coriander seeds, not only enhances flavor but also introduces potential digestive benefits.

Versatile Pairing: These turmeric cauliflower pickles are a versatile addition to various dishes, bringing both flavor and a nutritional boost.

Zesty Pickled Green Beans

Description: These zesty pickled green beans add a burst of tangy flavor and crispness to your palate. Whether enjoyed as a standalone snack or as a lively addition to salads and charcuterie boards, these pickled green beans are a delightful treat.

Preparation Time: 15 minutes

Cook Time: 10 minutes

Servings: 8

Ingredients:

1 pound of fresh green beans, trimmed

2 cups of white vinegar

1 cup of water

2 tablespoons pickling salt

1 tablespoon of sugar

2 cloves of garlic, peeled and sliced

1 teaspoon whole black peppercorns

1 teaspoon crushed red pepper flakes

2 sprigs of fresh dill

Instructions:

Trim the ends of the green beans to fit the height of your sterilized jars.

In a saucepan, combine white vinegar, water, pickling salt, sugar, garlic, black peppercorns, and red pepper flakes. Bring everything to a boil, stirring until the sugar and salt dissolve.

Pack the green beans vertically into sterilized jars, placing a sprig of fresh dill in each jar.

Pour the hot brine over the green beans, ensuring they are fully submerged and leaving about 1/2 inch of headspace.

Seal the jars and process them in a hot water bath for traditional canning. Allow the pickled green beans to rest for at least 2 weeks in a cool, dark place for optimal flavor development. Alternatively, refrigerate for at least 24 hours for a quicker infusion.

Health Benefits:

Nutrient-rich Green Beans: Green beans are a low-calorie vegetable rich in vitamins C and K, as well as fiber.

Garlic's Potential Health Benefits: Garlic may contribute to cardiovascular health and provide immune system support.

Peppercorns and Red Pepper Flakes: These spices not only add heat but may have potential digestive benefits.

Dill Infusion: Fresh dill not only enhances flavor but may also offer antioxidant and anti-inflammatory properties.

Pickled Red Onion Bliss

Description: Elevate your dishes with the vibrant and tangy goodness of pickled red onions. This quick and easy recipe adds a burst of flavor to salads, tacos, and more. Perfect for beginners and seasoned cooks alike, this pickling adventure promises a delightful addition to your culinary repertoire.

Preparation Time: 15 minutes

Pickling time: 24 hours

Ingredients:

2 medium-sized red onions, thinly sliced
1 cup apple cider vinegar
1 cup of water
2 tablespoons of sugar
1 ½ teaspoons salt
Optional: 1 teaspoon whole black peppercorns, 1-2 bay leaves

Instructions:

Prepare the onions.

Peel and thinly slice the red onions. Separate the slices into individual rings for even pickling.

Create the pickling liquid:

In a saucepan, combine the apple cider vinegar, water, sugar, and salt. Optionally, add black peppercorns and bay leaves for additional flavor complexity.

Bring to a simmer:

Over medium heat, bring the pickling liquid to a simmer. Stir until the sugar and salt dissolves completely.

Pack the jars:

Place the sliced red onions into sterilized glass jars. Ensure the jars are heat-resistant.

Pour the pickling liquid.

Carefully pour the hot pickling liquid over the red onions, ensuring they are fully submerged. Leave 1/2 inch headspace at the top.

Cool and Seal:

let the jars cool down to room temperature before sealing them. Once cooled, store the jars in the refrigerator for at least 24 hours to enhance the flavors.

Serve and enjoy:

Your pickled red onions are ready to amplify the taste of your favorite dishes. Add them to salads, sandwiches, or tacos for a delightful culinary experience.

Tips for beginners:

Experiment with the pickling liquid by adjusting the sugar and salt levels to suit your taste preferences. Customize the flavor profile by adding spices like cumin seeds or coriander for a unique twist.

Benefits:

Pickled red onions not only enhance the taste of your meals but also offer a vibrant color and a dose of probiotics.

Experience the joy of homemade pickled red onions—a simple yet versatile addition to your kitchen creations.

Pickled Jalapeño Slices

Description: Elevate your dishes with the zesty kick of pickled jalapeño slices. Perfect for adding a spicy punch to tacos, nachos, burgers, or any culinary creation that craves a touch of heat.

Preparation Time: 15 minutes

Cook Time: 10 minutes

Servings: 8

Ingredients:

1 pound of fresh jalapeños, thinly sliced

2 cups of white vinegar

1 cup of water

2 tablespoons pickling salt

1 tablespoon of sugar

3 cloves of garlic, peeled and sliced

1 teaspoon of whole cumin seeds

1 teaspoon of coriander seeds

1 teaspoon of black peppercorns

Instructions:

Prepare Jalapeños:

Wear gloves while slicing fresh jalapeños into thin rounds.

Prepare pickling liquid:

In a saucepan, combine white vinegar, water, pickling salt, sugar, garlic, cumin seeds, coriander seeds, and black peppercorns.

Bring everything in the pan to a boil over medium heat, stirring until the sugar and salt dissolve.

Pack the jars:

Pack the sliced jalapeños into sterilized jars, distributing the spices evenly.

Pour hot pickling liquid:

Cover the jalapenos in the hot pickling liquid ensuring they are fully submerged. Leave about 1/2 inch of headspace.

Seal the Jars:

Use a wet, damp cloth to wipe the rims and rim areas of the jars. Cover the jars with the sterilized lids, and screw on the bands until fingertip-tight.

Process for Canning (Optional):

If you're canning, process the jars in a hot water bath for 10 minutes for a secure seal.

Storage:

Allow the pickled jalapeño slices to cool to room temperature.

Store the jars in a cool, dark place for at least 2 weeks for optimal flavor development.

Alternatively, refrigerate for at least 24 hours for a quicker infusion.

Tips for beginners:

Use Gloves: Wear gloves while handling jalapeños to avoid irritation from the oils.

Balance Heat: Adjust the spice level by removing seeds for milder pickles or keeping them for extra heat.

Experiment with Spices: Customize the flavor profile by experimenting with additional spices like oregano or thyme.

Health Benefits:

Vitamin C Boost: Jalapeños are rich in vitamin C, contributing to immune health.

Metabolism Boost: The heat from jalapeños may temporarily increase metabolism.

Low-Calorie Flavor: Pickled jalapeños add bold flavor to dishes with minimal calories.

Mustard seed-pickled cabbage

Description: Transform humble cabbage into a tangy delight with this mustard seed pickling recipe. Enjoy it as a zesty side dish or elevate sandwiches and wraps with its crunchy texture and bold flavor.

Preparation Time: 15 minutes

Cook Time: 10 minutes

Servings: 8

Ingredients:

1 green cabbage(small head) thinly shredded

2 cups of white vinegar

1 cup of water

2 tablespoons pickling salt

2 tablespoons of mustard seeds

1 tablespoon of sugar

3 cloves of garlic, peeled and sliced

1 teaspoon turmeric powder (optional, for color)

Instructions:

Prepare Cabbage:

Remove the outer leaves of the cabbage and thinly shred the remaining head.

Prepare pickling liquid:

In a saucepan, combine white vinegar, water, pickling salt, mustard seeds, sugar, garlic, and turmeric powder, if using.

Bring everything in the pan to a boil over medium heat, stirring until the sugar and salt dissolve.

Pack the jars:

Pack the shredded cabbage into sterilized jars, distributing mustard seeds and garlic evenly.

Pour hot pickling liquid:

Cover the cabbage with the hot pickling liquid, ensuring it is fully submerged. Leave about 1/2 inch of headspace.

Seal the Jars:

Use a clean, damp cloth to wipe the rims and rim areas of the jars. Cover the jars with the sterilized lids, and screw on the bands until fingertip-tight.

Process for Canning (Optional):

If canning, process the jars in a hot water bath for 10 minutes for a secure seal.

Storage:

Allow the mustard seed-pickled cabbage to cool to room temperature.

Store the jars in a cool, dark place for at least 2 weeks for optimal flavor development.

Alternatively, refrigerate for at least 24 hours for a quicker infusion.

Tips for beginners:

Shred Evenly: Aim for uniform shredding of cabbage for consistent texture in your pickles.

Balance Salt and Sugar: Adjust the pickling salt and sugar to achieve a pleasing balance of tanginess and sweetness.

Experiment with Turmeric: Add turmeric for a vibrant color; adjust the quantity based on preference.

Health Benefits:

Cabbage Nutrients: Cabbage is rich in vitamins and antioxidants.

Mustard Seeds for Flavor: Mustard seeds add a distinct flavor and may offer anti-inflammatory benefits.

Gut-Friendly: Fermented cabbage contributes to gut health, providing probiotics for digestion.

CHAPTER 5: PICKLED FRUIT RECIPES

Pickled Mango Slices

Description: Immerse your taste buds in a tropical symphony with these naturally sweet and tangy pickled mango slices. Their vibrant flavor makes them a versatile addition to salads, grilled dishes, or a delightful standalone snack.

Preparation Time: 20 minutes

Cook Time: 10 minutes

Servings: 6

Ingredients:

3 large, ripe mangoes, peeled and sliced

1 cup of white vinegar

1/2 cup of water

1 tablespoon salt

1 teaspoon of mustard seeds

1 teaspoon whole black peppercorns

2 cloves of garlic, peeled and sliced

1 cinnamon stick

1 teaspoon of red pepper flakes for heat (optional)

Fresh mint leaves for garnish

Instructions:

Prepare Mangoes:

Peel and slice the ripe mangoes into thin, uniform slices.

Prepare pickling liquid:

In a saucepan, combine white vinegar, water, salt, mustard seeds, black peppercorns, garlic, cinnamon stick, and red pepper flakes if using.

Bring everything in the pan to a gentle boil over medium heat, stirring occasionally.

Pack the jars:

Pack the mango slices into sterilized jars, layering them with the prepared pickling liquid and spices.

Pour hot pickling liquid:

Cover the mango slices in the hot pickling liquid, ensuring they are fully immersed. Leave about 1/2 inch of headspace.

Seal the Jars:

Use a clean, damp cloth to wipe the rims and rim areas of the jars. Cover the jars with the sterilized lids, and screw on the bands until fingertip-tight.

Cooling and Infusion:

Let the jars cool to room temperature before refrigerating.

Let the pickled mango slices marinate for at least 24 hours to achieve optimal flavor.

Garnish and serve:

Before serving, garnish with fresh mint leaves for a burst of color and added freshness.

Tips for beginners:

Choose Ripe Mangoes: Select ripe mangoes for a naturally sweet and flavorful outcome.

Adjust Sweetness: As mangoes are sweet, feel free to omit or reduce sugar based on personal preference.

Experiment with heat: Add red pepper flakes for a hint of spice, adjusting to your desired level.

Health Benefits:

Rich in antioxidants: Mangoes are packed with antioxidants, supporting overall health.

Digestive Aid: Garlic and peppercorns contribute to digestive health.

Probiotic Boost: Fermented foods promote a healthy gut by providing beneficial probiotics.

Enjoy a delightful burst of tropical flavors with these homemade pickled mango slices!

Ginger-spiced pickled peaches

Description: Experience the perfect blend of sweetness and warmth with these ginger-spiced pickled peaches. A versatile addition to charcuterie boards, desserts, or enjoyed on their own.

Preparation Time: 20 minutes

Cook Time: 10 minutes

Servings: 6

Ingredients:

4 large peaches, peeled, pitted, and sliced

1 cup apple cider vinegar

1/2 cup of water

1 cup granulated sugar (optional)

1 tablespoon salt

1 tablespoon fresh ginger, grated

1 teaspoon whole cloves

1 teaspoon of cinnamon sticks

2 teaspoons black tea leaves (optional, for depth)

Fresh basil leaves for garnish

Instructions:

Prepare Peaches:

Peel, pit, and slice the peaches into uniform pieces.

Prepare pickling liquid:

In a saucepan, combine apple cider vinegar, water, sugar, salt, grated ginger, cloves, cinnamon sticks, and black tea leaves, if using.

Bring everything in the pan to a gentle boil over medium heat, stirring until the sugar and salt dissolve.

Pack the jars:

Pack the peach slices into sterilized jars, layering them with the pickling liquid and spices.

Pour hot pickling liquid:

Pour the hot pickling liquid over the peaches, ensuring they are fully immersed. Leave about 1/2 inch of headspace.

Seal the Jars:

Use a clean damp cloth to wipe the rims and rim areas of the jars. with a clean, damp cloth. Cover the jars with the sterilized lids and screw on the bands until fingertip-tight.

Cooling and Infusion:

Let the jars cool to room temperature before refrigerating.

Let the ginger-spiced pickled peaches marinate for at least 24 hours to enhance their flavor.

Garnish and serve:

Before serving, garnish with fresh basil leaves for an aromatic touch.

Tips for beginners:

Choose Ripe Peaches: Opt for ripe peaches for a naturally sweet and juicy outcome.

Adjust Sweetness: Tailor the sweetness to your preference by modifying the sugar quantity.

Experiment with Tea: Black tea leaves add depth; adjust the quantity based on preference.

Health Benefits:

Peach Nutrients: Peaches offer vitamins, minerals, and antioxidants.

Anti-Inflammatory: Ginger provides potential anti-inflammatory benefits.

Enjoy the delightful fusion of sweetness and spice with these homemade ginger-spiced pickled peaches!

Lemon and rosemary pickled strawberries

Description: Elevate your taste buds with the refreshing blend of citrus and herbal notes in these lemon and rosemary pickled strawberries. Perfect for topping desserts, salads, or enjoying as a unique standalone treat.

Preparation Time: 15 minutes

Cook Time: 5 minutes

Servings: 4

Ingredients:

2 cups fresh strawberries, hulled and halved

1/2 cup white balsamic vinegar

1/4 cup of water

1/4 cup honey

Zest of 1 lemon

Juice of 1 lemon

2 sprigs of fresh rosemary

1/2 teaspoon black peppercorns

1/4 teaspoon sea salt

Instructions:

Prepare Strawberries:

Hull and halve the fresh strawberries.

Prepare pickling liquid:

In a saucepan, combine white balsamic vinegar, water, honey, lemon zest, lemon juice, rosemary sprigs, black peppercorns, and sea salt.

Bring everything in the pan to a gentle boil over medium heat, stirring until the honey dissolves.

Pack the jars:

Pack the strawberry halves into sterilized jars, ensuring an even distribution of rosemary and peppercorns.

Pour hot pickling liquid:

Pour the hot pickling liquid over the strawberries, making sure they are fully immersed. Leave about 1/2 inch of headspace.

Seal the Jars:

Use a clean, damp cloth to wipe the rims and rim areas of the jars. Cover the jars with the sterilized lids, and screw on the bands until fingertip-tight.

Cooling and Infusion:

Let the jars cool to room temperature before keeping in the refrigerator.

Let the lemon and rosemary pickled strawberries marinate for at least 4 hours for optimal flavor.

Serve and enjoy:

Spoon these delightful pickled strawberries over desserts or salads, or savor them on their own.

Tips for beginners:

Choose Ripe Strawberries: Opt for ripe strawberries for enhanced sweetness.

Adjust Sweetness: Modify honey quantity to achieve your preferred level of sweetness.

Experiment with Zest: Lemon zest adds a burst of citrusy flavor; adjust to taste.

Health Benefits:

Strawberry Nutrients: Strawberries offer vitamins, antioxidants, and fiber.

Digestive Aid: Lemon and rosemary may contribute to digestive health.

Delight in the unique flavors of lemon and rosemary with these homemade pickled strawberries!

Vanilla Bean Pickled Pears

Description: Immerse yourself in the delightful combination of sweet and aromatic flavors with these vanilla bean pickled pears. A versatile addition to desserts, cheese boards, or enjoyed on their own.

Preparation Time: 20 minutes

Cook Time: 15 minutes

Servings: 6

Ingredients:

4 large, ripe but firm pears, peeled, cored, and sliced

1 cup white wine vinegar

1/2 cup of water

1 cup granulated sugar

1 vanilla bean, split and scraped

1 cinnamon stick

4 whole cloves

1/2 teaspoon black peppercorns

Pinch of salt

Instructions:

Prepare Pears:

Peel, core, and slice the ripe but firm pears.

Prepare pickling liquid:

In a saucepan, combine white wine vinegar, water, granulated sugar, vanilla bean (both seeds and pod), cinnamon stick, cloves, black peppercorns, and a pinch of salt.

Bring everything in the pan to a gentle boil over medium heat, stirring until the sugar dissolves.

Pack the jars:

Pack the pear slices into sterilized jars, ensuring an even distribution of vanilla seeds and spices.

Pour hot pickling liquid:

Pour the hot pickling liquid over the pear slices, making sure they are fully immersed. Leave about 1/2 inch of headspace.

Seal the Jars:

Use a clean, damp cloth to wipe the rims and rim areas of the jars. Cover the jars with the sterilized lids, and screw on the bands until fingertip-tight.

Cooling and Infusion:

Let the jars cool to room temperature before keeping them in the refrigerator for quick pickling.

Let the vanilla bean pickled pears marinate for at least 24 hours for optimal flavor.

Serve and enjoy.

Enjoy these flavorful pickled pears on their own or as a delightful accompaniment to desserts and cheese boards.

Tips for beginners:

Choose Firm Pears: Select ripe but firm pears for a satisfying texture.

Adjust Sugar Levels: Tailor the sweetness by modifying the sugar quantity based on preference.

Reuse Vanilla Pod: After pickling, rinse the vanilla pod and use it to infuse sugar for other culinary endeavors.

Health Benefits:

Pear Nutrients: Pears are rich in fiber, vitamins, and antioxidants.

Aromatic Vanilla: Vanilla may have calming and antioxidant properties.

Cinnamon-Spiced Pickled Apples

Description: Indulge in the warm and cozy flavors of cinnamon-spiced pickled apples. This versatile pickle adds a touch of autumn to your dishes—perfect for pairing with desserts, salads, or enjoying as a flavorful snack.

Preparation Time: 15 minutes

Cook Time: 10 minutes

Servings: 4

Ingredients:

4 medium-sized apples, cored and sliced

1 cup apple cider vinegar

1/2 cup of water

1 cup brown sugar

2 cinnamon sticks

4 whole cloves

1/2 teaspoon whole allspice

Pinch of salt

Instructions:

Prepare Apples:

Core and slice the medium-sized apples.

Prepare pickling liquid:

In a saucepan, combine apple cider vinegar, water, brown sugar, cinnamon sticks, cloves, whole allspice, and a pinch of salt.

Bring everything in the pan to a gentle boil over medium heat, stirring until the sugar dissolves.

Pack the jars:

Pack the apple slices into sterilized jars, ensuring an even distribution of spices.

Pour hot pickling liquid:

Pour the hot pickling liquid over the apple slices, ensuring they are fully immersed. Leave about 1/2 inch of headspace.

Seal the Jars:

Use a clean damp cloth to wipe the rims and rim areas of the jars. Cover the jars with the sterilized lids and screw on the bands until fingertip-tight.

Cooling and Infusion:

Allow the jars to cool to room temperature before keeping in the refrigerator.

Let the cinnamon-spiced pickled apples marinate for at least 24 hours for optimal flavor.

Serve and enjoy:

Pair these delightful pickled apples with desserts, incorporate them into salads, or relish them as a sweet and spiced snack.

Tips for beginners:

Apple Variety Matters: Choose a firm apple variety suitable for pickling, such as Granny Smith or Honeycrisp.

Adjust Sweetness: Modify the brown sugar quantity to achieve the desired level of sweetness.

Reuse Spices: After pickling, strain and reuse the cinnamon sticks, cloves, and allspice for other culinary creations.

Health Benefits:

Apple Nutrients: Apples are a good source of fiber, vitamins, and antioxidants.

Digestive Aid: Cinnamon and cloves may offer digestive benefits.

Cardamom-infused pickled plums

Description: Elevate your culinary experience with the exotic fragrance of cardamom-infused pickled plums. This delightful pickle pairs exceptionally well with cheese boards, desserts, or as a unique addition to your favorite dishes.

Preparation Time: 20 minutes

Cook Time: 15 minutes

Servings: 6

Ingredients:

2 cups ripe plums, pitted and halved

1 cup of red wine vinegar

1/2 cup of water

1 cup granulated sugar

4-5 cardamom pods, lightly crushed

1 teaspoon whole black peppercorns

Pinch of salt

Instructions:

Prepare Plums:

Pit and halve the ripe plums.

Prepare pickling liquid:

In a saucepan, combine red wine vinegar, water, granulated sugar, crushed cardamom pods, black peppercorns, and a pinch of salt.

Bring everything in the pan to a gentle boil over medium heat, stirring until the sugar dissolves.

Pack the jars:

Pack the plum halves into sterilized jars, ensuring an even distribution of cardamom and peppercorns.

Pour hot pickling liquid:

Pour the hot pickling liquid over the plum halves, ensuring they are fully immersed. Leave about 1/2 inch of headspace.

Seal the Jars:

Use a clean, damp cloth to wipe the rims and rim areas of the jars. Cover the jars with the sterilized lids, and screw on the bands until fingertip-tight.

Cooling and Infusion:

Allow the jars to cool to room temperature before placing them in the refrigerator.

Let the cardamom-infused pickled plums marinate for at least 24 hours for optimal flavor.

Serve and enjoy.

Delight in the aromatic essence of cardamom-infused pickled plums alongside cheeses, desserts, or as a unique flavor enhancer in your favorite dishes.

Tips for beginners:

Select Ripe Plums: Choose plums that are ripe but still firm for a satisfying texture.

Adjust Sugar Levels: Modify the sugar quantity based on your desired level of sweetness.

Experiment with Cardamom: Add more or less cardamom based on your preference for this exotic spice.

Health Benefits:

Plum Nutrients: Plums are rich in vitamins, antioxidants, and fiber.

Cardamom Essence: Cardamom may offer digestive and antioxidant benefits.

Savor the enchanting blend of cardamom-infused pickled plums in this easy-to-follow recipe!

Cherry and Basil Pickles

Description: Immerse your taste buds in the vibrant harmony of cherries and basil with this delightful pickle. Perfect for adding a burst of flavor to salads, desserts, or enjoyed on its own as a refreshing treat.

Preparation Time: 15 minutes

Cook Time: 10 minutes

Servings: 4

Ingredients:

2 cups fresh cherries, pitted and halved

1 cup apple cider vinegar

1/2 cup of water

1/2 cup honey

1 handful of fresh basil leaves

1 teaspoon of black peppercorns

Pinch of salt

Instructions:

Prepare Cherries:

Pit and halve the fresh cherries.

Prepare pickling liquid:

In a saucepan, combine apple cider vinegar, water, honey, fresh basil leaves, black peppercorns, and a pinch of salt.

Bring everything in the pan to a gentle boil over medium heat, stirring until the honey dissolves.

Pack the jars:

Pack the halved cherries into sterilized jars, distributing basil leaves and peppercorns evenly.

Pour hot pickling liquid:

Pour the hot pickling liquid over the cherries, ensuring they are fully immersed. Leave about 1/2 inch of headspace.

Seal the Jars:

Use a clean, damp cloth to wipe the rims and rim areas of the jars. Cover the jars with the sterilized lids, and screw on the bands until fingertip-tight.

Cooling and Infusion:

Allow the jars to cool to room temperature before placing them in the refrigerator.

Let the cherry and basil pickles marinate for at least 24 hours for optimal flavor.

Serve and enjoy:

Experience the delightful combination of cherries and basil by incorporating this pickle into salads, desserts, or savoring it on its own.

Tips for beginners:

Fresh Cherries: Opt for ripe, fresh cherries for a burst of natural sweetness.

Adjust Honey Quantity: Modify the honey quantity based on your preference for sweetness.

Explore Basil Varieties: Experiment with different basil varieties for unique flavor profiles.

Health Benefits:

Cherry Nutrients: Cherries are rich in antioxidants, vitamins, and anti-inflammatory compounds.

Basil Freshness: Basil adds freshness and may offer anti-inflammatory properties.

Delight in the delightful fusion of cherries and basil with this easy-to-follow pickle recipe!

Citrusy Pickled Watermelon Rind

Description: Transform watermelon rind into a zesty and citrusy delight with this unique pickle. The infusion of citrus flavors makes it a refreshing accompaniment to summer dishes, salads, or as a standalone treat.

Preparation Time: 20 minutes

Cook Time: 15 minutes

Servings: 6

Ingredients:

4 cups watermelon rind, peeled and chopped into bite-sized pieces

1 cup of white vinegar

1 cup of water

1 cup granulated sugar

Zest of 1 lemon

Zest of 1 orange

1 cinnamon stick

1 teaspoon whole cloves

Pinch of salt

Instructions:

Prepare the watermelon rinse:

Peel the watermelon rind and cut it into bite-sized pieces.

Prepare pickling liquid:

In a saucepan, combine white vinegar, water, granulated sugar, lemon zest, orange zest, cinnamon stick, whole cloves, and a pinch of salt.

Bring everything in the pan to a gentle boil over medium heat, stirring until the sugar dissolves.

Pack the jars:

Pack the watermelon rind pieces into sterilized jars, ensuring an even distribution of citrus zest, cinnamon, and cloves.

Pour hot pickling liquid:

Pour the hot pickling liquid over the watermelon rind, ensuring all pieces are fully submerged. Leave about 1/2 inch of headspace.

Seal the Jars:

Use a clean, damp cloth to wipe the rims and rim areas of the jars. Cover the jars with the sterilized lids, and screw on the bands until fingertip-tight.

Cooling and Infusion:

Allow the jars to cool to room temperature before placing them in the refrigerator.

Let the citrusy pickled watermelon rind infuse for at least 24 hours for optimal flavor.

Serve and enjoy:

Experience a refreshing burst of citrus with this pickled watermelon rind. Perfect for adding a unique twist to summer dishes or enjoyed on its own.

Tips for beginners:

Uniform Cutting: Cut the watermelon rind into uniform, bite-sized pieces for consistent texture.

Adjust Sugar Levels: Modify the sugar quantity based on your preferred level of sweetness.

Experiment with Citrus Zest: Explore different citrus zest combinations for varied flavor profiles.

Health Benefits:

Watermelon Rind Nutrients: Watermelon rind is a good source of vitamins and antioxidants.

Citrus Zest Freshness: Citrus zest adds a burst of freshness and may provide additional nutritional benefits.

Enjoy the citrusy goodness of pickled watermelon rind in this easy-to-follow recipe!

Kiwi and Mint Pickle

Description: Embark on a flavor journey with this delightful kiwi and mint pickle. The combination of sweet kiwi and refreshing mint creates a unique and tangy pickle perfect for adding a twist to desserts, salads, or as a palate cleanser.

Preparation Time: 15 minutes

Cook Time: 10 minutes

Servings: 4

Ingredients:

2 cups ripe Kiwi, peeled and diced

1 cup of white vinegar

1/2 cup of water

1/2 cup granulated sugar

1/4 cup fresh mint leaves, finely chopped

1 teaspoon whole black peppercorns

Pinch of salt

Instructions:

Prepare Kiwi:

Peel and dice the ripe kiwi.

Prepare pickling liquid:

In a saucepan, combine white vinegar, water, granulated sugar, chopped mint leaves, whole black peppercorns, and a pinch of salt.

Bring everything in the pan to a gentle boil over medium heat, stirring until the sugar dissolves.

Pack the jars:

Pack the diced kiwi into sterilized jars, ensuring an even distribution of mint and peppercorns.

Pour hot pickling liquid:

Pour the hot pickling liquid over the kiwi, ensuring all pieces are fully immersed. Leave about 1/2 inch of headspace.

Seal the Jars:

Use a clean, damp cloth to wipe the rims and rim areas of the jars. Cover the jars with the sterilized lids, and screw on the bands until fingertip-tight.

Cooling and Infusion:

Allow the jars to cool to room temperature before placing them in the refrigerator.

Let the kiwi and mint pickles infuse for at least 24 hours for optimal flavor.

Serve and enjoy:

Indulge in the delightful combination of sweet kiwi and fresh mint. Ideal for enhancing desserts, salads, or as a palate-cleansing treat.

Tips for beginners:

Ripe Kiwi Selection: Choose ripe kiwi for a naturally sweet flavor.

Adjust Sugar Levels: Modify the sugar quantity based on your desired level of sweetness.

Mint Infusion: Experiment with the intensity of mint flavor by adjusting the quantity to your preference.

Health Benefits:

Kiwi Nutrients: Kiwi is rich in vitamin C, fiber, and antioxidants.

Mint Freshness: Mint adds a refreshing element and may aid digestion.

Savor the unique blend of kiwi and mint in this easy-to-follow pickle recipe!

Pineapple and Jalapeño Pickle

Description: Elevate your taste buds with the perfect balance of sweetness and heat in this pineapple and jalapeño pickle. Ideal for adding a spicy kick to tacos, sandwiches, or enjoyed as a standalone treat.

Preparation Time: 20 minutes

Cook Time: 15 minutes

Servings: 6

Ingredients:

2 cups fresh pineapple, diced

2 jalapeño peppers, sliced (seeds removed for milder heat)

1 cup of white vinegar

1/2 cup of water

1/2 cup granulated sugar

1 teaspoon of whole coriander seeds

1/2 teaspoon cumin seeds

Pinch of salt

Instructions:

Prepare pineapple and jalapeños:

Dice fresh pineapple and slice jalapeño peppers, removing seeds for milder heat.

Prepare pickling liquid:

In a saucepan, combine white vinegar, water, granulated sugar, coriander seeds, cumin seeds, and a pinch of salt.

Bring everything in the pan to a gentle boil over medium heat, stirring until the sugar dissolves.

Pack the jars:

Pack the diced pineapple and sliced jalapeños into sterilized jars, distributing seeds and spices evenly.

Pour hot pickling liquid:

Pour the hot pickling liquid over the pineapple and jalapeños, ensuring all pieces are fully submerged. Leave about 1/2 inch of headspace.

Seal the Jars:

Use a clean, damp cloth to wipe the rims and rim areas of the jars. Cover the jars with the sterilized lids, and screw on the bands until fingertip-tight.!.

Cooling and Infusion:

Allow the jars to cool to room temperature before placing them in the refrigerator.

Let the pineapple and jalapeño pickles infuse for at least 24 hours for optimal flavor.

Serve and enjoy:

Experience the perfect blend of sweet pineapple and spicy jalapeños. It is ideal for spicing up tacos, sandwiches, or enjoying it on its own.

Tips for beginners:

Adjust Jalapeño Heat: Control the heat level by adjusting the quantity of jalapeños and removing seeds.

Experiment with Spices: Customize the flavor profile by experimenting with different spices like black pepper or chili flakes.

Fresh Pineapple: Opt for fresh, ripe pineapple for the best natural sweetness.

Health Benefits:

Pineapple Nutrients: Pineapple is rich in vitamin C, manganese, and antioxidants.

Jalapeño Heat: Jalapeños may boost metabolism and provide a dose of capsaicin, known for its potential health benefits.

CHAPTER 6: FERMENTED VEGETABLE RECIPES

Classic Sauerkraut

Description: Experience the timeless delight of homemade sauerkraut with this classic recipe. Fermented to perfection, this tangy and crunchy sauerkraut is a versatile addition to sandwiches, salads, or enjoyed as a flavorful side dish.

Preparation Time: 20 minutes

Fermentation Time: 2 to 4 weeks

Servings: 8

Ingredients:

1 medium-sized green cabbage (about 2-3 pounds)

1 tablespoon sea salt (non-iodized)

Optional: Caraway seeds for added flavor

Instructions:

Prepare Cabbage:

Remove the outer leaves of the cabbage and reserve one or two.

Finely shred the cabbage using a knife or a mandoline.

Salt and Massage:

In a large mixing bowl, combine the shredded cabbage with sea salt.

Massage the salt into the cabbage using your hands for about 10 minutes until it starts to release its juices.

Pack the Jar:

Pack the salted cabbage tightly into a clean, wide-mouth glass jar, layering it as you go.

Press down firmly to ensure the cabbage is submerged in its juices.

Add optional caraway seeds:

If desired, sprinkle caraway seeds between the layers for an additional layer of flavor.

Cover with Reserved Leaves:

Place one or two reserved cabbage leaves on top to keep the shredded cabbage submerged.

Weight Down and Cover:

Place a fermentation weight or a clean, sanitized stone on top of the cabbage to keep it submerged.

Cover the jar loosely with a lid to allow gasses to escape during fermentation.

Fermentation:

Allow the sauerkraut to ferment at room temperature for 2 to 4 weeks, depending on taste preferences.

Check periodically, pressing the cabbage down if it rises above the liquid.

Taste and Store:

Taste the sauerkraut, and when it reaches the desired tanginess, remove the weight and cabbage leaves.

Seal the jar with a tight lid and store it in the refrigerator for several months.

Serve and enjoy:

Incorporate this classic sauerkraut into sandwiches, salads, or savor its bold flavor as a side dish.

Tips for beginners:

Sanitization: Ensure all utensils and the jar are thoroughly sanitized to prevent unwanted bacteria.

Patience is key. Allow sufficient fermentation time for the best flavor and texture.

Health Benefits:

Probiotics: Sauerkraut is a natural source of probiotics, promoting gut health.

Vitamin C: Cabbage is rich in vitamin C, contributing to immune support.

Experience the art of fermentation with this simple yet delightful classic sauerkraut recipe!

Spicy Kimchi

Description: Embark on a flavorful journey with this spicy kimchi recipe, a staple in Korean cuisine. Packed with bold spices and fermented to perfection, this kimchi adds a fiery kick to rice bowls, tacos, or can be enjoyed on its own as a zesty side.

Preparation Time: 30 minutes

Fermentation Time: 1 to 2 weeks

Servings: 10

Ingredients:

1 napa cabbage (about 2 pounds)

1/4 cup sea salt (non-iodized)

1 tablespoon grated ginger

1 tablespoon minced garlic

2 tablespoons Korean red pepper flakes (gochugaru)

2 tablespoons of fish sauce or soy sauce if you are a vegetarian.

1 tablespoon of sugar

2 green onions, chopped

1 carrot, julienned

Instructions:

Prepare Cabbage:

Cut the napa cabbage in half lengthwise, then remove the core.

Chop the cabbage into bite-sized pieces.

Salt and Rest:

In a large bowl, sprinkle salt between the cabbage leaves, ensuring even distribution.

Allow the cabbage to rest for 1 to 2 hours, tossing occasionally.

Rinse and drain:

Rinse the cabbage thoroughly to get rid of excess salt.

Put the cabbage in a colander and allow it to drain for about 15 minutes.

Create Spice Paste:

In a separate bowl, mix grated ginger, minced garlic, Korean red pepper flakes, fish sauce (or soy sauce), and sugar to create a spice paste.

Combine cabbage and paste.

In a large mixing bowl, combine the drained cabbage, chopped green onions, julienned carrot, and the spice paste.

Wear gloves and massage the spice paste into the cabbage, ensuring an even coating.

Pack in Jars:

Pack the spiced cabbage mixture into clean, wide-mouth glass jars, pressing it down as you go.

Leave some headspace at the top.

Fermentation:

Seal the jars loosely so gasses can escape.

Allow the kimchi to ferment at room temperature for 1 to 2 weeks, depending on your desired level of fermentation.

Taste and refrigerate:

Taste the kimchi, and when it reaches your preferred level of fermentation, seal the jars tightly and refrigerate.

Serve and enjoy:

Add a spicy kick to various dishes or savor the zesty flavor of kimchi on its own.

Tips for beginners:

Adjust Spice Level: Control the heat by adjusting the amount of Korean red pepper flakes.

Gloves for Mixing: Wear gloves when massaging the spice paste to avoid irritation from the pepper flakes.

Health Benefits:

Probiotics: Kimchi is rich in probiotics, supporting digestive health.

Vitamins and Antioxidants: Cabbage and other vegetables in kimchi provide essential vitamins and antioxidants.

Delight in the bold and spicy flavors of homemade kimchi with this easy-to-follow recipe!

Tangy Dill Pickles

Description: Revel in the classic goodness of tangy dill pickles with this straightforward recipe. Bursting with the vibrant flavors of dill and garlic, these pickles are an ideal accompaniment to sandwiches, burgers, or enjoyed straight from the jar.

Preparation Time: 15 minutes

Fermentation Time: 1 to 2 weeks

Servings: 8

Ingredients:

2 pounds of pickled cucumbers

3 cups of water

1 cup white vinegar (5% acidity)

2 tablespoons pickling salt

2 teaspoons of dill seeds

4 garlic cloves, peeled

1 teaspoon of black peppercorns

1/2 teaspoon red pepper flakes (optional, for heat)

Fresh dill sprigs

Instructions:

Prepare Cucumbers:

Wash the pickling cucumbers thoroughly and trim off the blossom ends.

Cut the cucumbers into spears or leave them whole, depending on your preference.

Create Brine:

In a saucepan, combine water, white vinegar, and pickling salt.

Bring everything in the pan to a boil, stirring until the salt dissolves. Then let it cool to room temperature.

Pack Jars:

Pack the cucumber spears or whole cucumbers into sterilized jars.

Add dill seeds, garlic cloves, black peppercorns, red pepper flakes (if using), and fresh dill sprigs to each jar.

Pour Brine:

Pour the cooled brine over the cucumbers, leaving about 1/2 inch of headspace at the top of the jar.

Seal Jars:

Use a clean, damp cloth to wipe the rims and rim areas of the jars. Cover the jars with the sterilized lids, and screw on the bands until fingertip-tight.!

Fermentation:

Allow the pickles to ferment at room temperature for 1 to 2 weeks. Check periodically for your preferred level of tanginess.

Taste and Store:

Taste the pickles, and when they reach the desired tanginess, seal the jars tightly and store them in the refrigerator.

Serve and enjoy:

Add a burst of tangy freshness to your favorite dishes with these homemade dill pickles.

Tips for beginners:

Choose Fresh Cucumbers: Opt for fresh, firm cucumbers for crisp pickles.

Experiment with Spice: Adjust the red pepper flakes to control the level of heat in your pickles.

Health Benefits:

Low in Calories: Pickles are low-calorie snacks, making them a guilt-free addition to your diet.

Hydration: Cucumbers contribute to hydration, providing a water-rich crunch.

Indulge in the delightful tanginess of homemade dill pickles with this simple and flavorful recipe!

Garlic Lovers' Fermented Green Beans

Description: Elevate your snacking game with these garlic lovers' fermented green beans. Packed with the robust flavors of garlic and spices, these fermented green beans are a crunchy delight, perfect for solo munching or as a zesty addition to salads and appetizer platters.

Preparation Time: 20 minutes

Fermentation Time: 1 to 2 weeks

Servings: 6

Ingredients:

1 pound of fresh green beans, trimmed

2 cups of water

1 tablespoon pickling salt

4 cloves of garlic, peeled and sliced

1 teaspoon of black peppercorns

1 teaspoon red pepper flakes (adjust to taste)

1 teaspoon of mustard seeds

Fresh dill sprigs

Instructions:

Prepare green beans:

Wash and trim the fresh green beans to fit the height of your jars.

Create Brine:

In a saucepan, combine water and pickling salt. Bring everything in the pan to a boil, stirring until the salt dissolves, then let it cool to room temperature.

Pack Jars:

Pack the trimmed green beans into sterilized jars, standing them upright.

Add Flavorings:

Add sliced garlic, black peppercorns, red pepper flakes, mustard seeds, and fresh dill sprigs to each jar.

Pour Brine:

Pour the cooled brine over the green beans, they are fully submerged. At the top, leave a headspace of approximately 1/2 inch.

Seal Jars:

Use a clean, damp cloth to wipe the rims and rim areas of the jars. Cover the jars with the sterilized lids, and screw on the bands until fingertip-tight.

Fermentation:

Allow the green beans to ferment at room temperature for 1 to 2 weeks. Check periodically for your preferred level of fermentation.

Taste and refrigerate:

Taste the green beans, and when they reach the desired crunchiness and tanginess, seal the jars tightly and store them in the refrigerator.

Serve and enjoy.

Savor the bold garlic-infused flavor of these fermented green beans as a standalone snack or paired with your favorite dishes.

Tips for beginners:

Consistent Trim: Trim green beans to a consistent height for even fermentation.

Adjust Spice Level: Customize the heat by adjusting the amount of red pepper flakes.

Health Benefits:

Fiber-Rich Snack: Green beans are a good source of dietary fiber, promoting digestive health.

Probiotic Boost: Fermented green beans contribute to a healthy gut with beneficial probiotics.

Experience the garlicky goodness of homemade fermented green beans with this easy-to-follow and flavorful recipe!

Carrot and Ginger Ferment

Description: Delight your taste buds with the vibrant combination of sweet carrots and zesty ginger in this carrot and ginger ferment. Perfect for adding a burst of flavor to salads, wraps, or enjoyed on its own, this ferment offers a crunchy and tangy experience with every bite.

Preparation Time: 15 minutes

Fermentation Time: 1 to 2 weeks

Servings: 4

Ingredients:

1 pound of carrots, peeled and cut into matchsticks
2 cups of water
1 tablespoon pickling salt
1 tablespoon fresh ginger, grated
2 cloves garlic, minced
1 teaspoon of coriander seeds
1 teaspoon of mustard seeds
Fresh cilantro leaves (optional, for garnish)

Instructions:

Prepare Carrots:

Peel and cut the carrots into matchsticks or thin strips.

Create Brine:

In a saucepan, combine water and pickling salt. Bring everything in the pan to a boil, stirring until the salt dissolves. Then let it cool to room temperature.

Pack Jars:

Pack the carrot matchsticks into sterilized jars, ensuring they are tightly packed.

Add Flavorings:

Add grated ginger, minced garlic, coriander seeds, and mustard seeds to each jar.

Pour Brine:

Pour the already prepared cool brine over the carrots, making sure they are fully submerged. Leave about 1/2 inch of headspace.

Seal Jars:

Use a clean, damp cloth to wipe the rims and rim areas of the jars. Cover the jars with the sterilized lids, and screw on the bands until fingertip-tight.!

Fermentation:

Allow the carrot and ginger to ferment at room temperature for 1 to 2 weeks. Taste periodically for your desired level of fermentation.

Garnish and refrigerate:

If desired, garnish with fresh cilantro leaves before sealing the jars.
Once the desired fermentation is achieved, store the jars in the refrigerator.

Serve and enjoy:

Enjoy the crisp texture and tangy flavor of this carrot and ginger ferment as a versatile addition to your meals.

Tips for beginners:

Uniform Cutting: Aim for uniform matchstick sizes for even fermentation.
Adjust Ginger: Customize the ginger intensity based on personal preference.

Health Benefits:

Rich in antioxidants: Carrots are packed with antioxidants that promote overall health.
Ginger's Digestive Aid: Ginger contributes to digestive health, providing relief from nausea and aiding digestion.

Savor the dynamic flavors of carrot and ginger fermentation, a delightful addition to your fermented food repertoire!

Beet Kvass

Description: Immerse yourself in the world of fermented beverages with the rich and earthy notes of Beet Kvass. This drink, crafted from the simplicity of beets, offers a unique blend of flavors and a natural touch of sweetness. Beyond its refreshing taste, Beet Kvass brings the added benefit of probiotics, making it a delightful and healthy addition to your beverage repertoire.

Preparation Time: 15 minutes

Fermentation Time: 7 to 14 days

Servings: 4

Ingredients:

2 medium-sized beets, peeled and cubed

1 tablespoon sea salt

1 tablespoon whey (optional)

Filtered water

Fresh ginger slices (optional, for added flavor)

Instructions:

Prepare Beets:

Peel and cube the beets into small, bite-sized pieces.

Create Brine:

In a large, sterilized jar, add the beet cubes and sea salt.

If using whey, add it to the jar.

Fill with water.

Pour filtered water into the jar, leaving about an inch of headspace.

Add ginger (optional):

If desired, add fresh ginger slices to enhance the flavor.

Mix and seal:

Gently stir the ingredients in the jar to dissolve the salt.

Seal the jar with a lid, ensuring it's airtight.

Fermentation:

Allow the jar to ferment at room temperature for 7 to 14 days. Check for the desired flavor strength.

Strain and refrigerate:

Once fermented, strain the liquid into a clean bottle, discarding the beet cubes.

Refrigerate the Beet Kvass for a chilled and ready-to-enjoy beverage.

Serve and enjoy:

Pour a glass of Beet Kvass over ice, savoring the unique taste and the natural effervescence.

Tips for beginners:

Be Mindful of Fermentation Time: Taste your beet kvass periodically during fermentation to find the right balance between sweetness and tanginess.

Experiment with Ginger: If you enjoy a hint of warmth, try adding ginger slices to your Beet Kvass for a delightful twist.

Quality Ingredients Matter: Choose fresh, organic beets for the best flavor and nutrient content.

Health Benefits:

Probiotic Boost: Beet Kvass is a natural source of probiotics, supporting a healthy gut microbiome.

Rich in Nutrients: Beets contain essential vitamins and minerals, including folate, potassium, and vitamin C.

Hydration with Flavor: Enjoy the hydrating properties of Beet Kvass with a flavor profile that stands out from typical beverages.

Sip and savor the goodness of Beet Kvass, a simple yet impactful addition to your fermented beverage choices.

Radish and Turnip Ferment

Description: Elevate your palate with the crisp and zesty combination of radish and turnip ferment. This ferment offers a delightful crunch and a burst of natural flavors that make it a versatile companion to salads, sandwiches, or a simple snack.

Preparation Time: 20 minutes

Fermentation Time: 7 to 10 days

Servings: 4

Ingredients:

1 bunch of radishes, thinly sliced

2 small turnips, peeled and julienned

1 tablespoon sea salt

1 teaspoon of mustard seeds

2 cloves garlic, minced

1 teaspoon dill seeds (optional)

Filtered water

Instructions:

Prepare Vegetables:

Wash and thinly slice radishes.

Peel and julienne turnips.

Create Brine:

In a large, sterilized jar, combine radishes, turnips, sea salt, mustard seeds, garlic, and dill seeds if using.

Pack the Jar:

Tightly pack the vegetables into the jar, leaving about an inch of headspace.

Fill with water.

Pour filtered water into the jar, ensuring the vegetables are fully submerged.

Mix and seal:

Gently stir the ingredients to dissolve the salt.

Seal the jar with an airtight lid.

Fermentation:

Let the jar ferment at room temperature for 7 to 10 days. Check for desired flavor and crunchiness.

Taste and refrigerate:

Taste a small portion to determine if the fermentation is complete.

Once satisfied, refrigerate the radish and turnips to halt the fermentation process.

Serve and enjoy:

Incorporate this ferment into salads, sandwiches, or enjoy it as a tangy snack.

Tips for beginners:

Consistent Slicing: Aim for uniform slicing for even fermentation and a consistent texture.

Experiment with Dill: Dill seeds add an extra layer of flavor; try it if you enjoy dill in your ferments.

Health Benefits:

Cruciferous Nutrition: Radishes and turnips belong to the cruciferous vegetable family, known for their nutrient density.

Digestive Support: Fermented vegetables provide probiotics that contribute to a healthy digestive system.

Discover the delightful union of radish and turnip fermentation, a crunchy and tangy addition to your fermented creations.

Cabbage and Caraway Kraut

Description: Immerse your taste buds in the harmonious blend of cabbage and caraway kraut. This classic ferment combines the simplicity of cabbage with the warm, earthy notes of caraway seeds, resulting in a kraut that pairs well with various dishes and adds a probiotic punch to your meals.

Preparation Time: 15 minutes

Fermentation Time: 10 to 14 days

Servings: 6

Ingredients:

1 small head of green cabbage, finely shredded

1 tablespoon sea salt

1 tablespoon caraway seeds

Filtered water

Instructions:

Prepare Cabbage:

Remove the outer leaves of the cabbage and finely shred the remaining head.

Create Brine:

In a large, sterilized bowl, combine shredded cabbage, sea salt, and caraway seeds.

Massage the mixture.

Use clean hands to massage the cabbage mixture thoroughly. This helps release the natural juices.

Pack the Jar:

Tightly pack the cabbage mixture into a sterilized jar, pressing it down to eliminate air pockets.

Cover with brine.

Pour any liquid released during massaging into the jar, ensuring the cabbage is fully submerged. If needed, add filtered water to cover.

Seal the Jar:

Seal the jar with an airtight lid, leaving some headspace to accommodate the expansion during fermentation.

Fermentation:

Let the jar ferment at room temperature for 10 to 14 days. Check for the desired tanginess.

Taste and refrigerate:

Taste a small portion to gauge the flavor. Once satisfied, refrigerate the kraut to slow down fermentation.

Serve and enjoy:

Incorporate cabbage and caraway kraut into sandwiches, salads, or enjoy it as a flavorful side dish.

Tips for beginners:

Even Shredding: Aim for uniform shredding to ensure consistent fermentation.

Adjust Salt: Feel free to adjust the salt quantity based on your taste preferences.

Health Benefits:

Probiotic Rich: This kraut is a probiotic powerhouse, contributing to a healthy gut microbiome.

Caraway Seed Goodness: Caraway seeds may aid digestion and add a unique flavor to the kraut.

Delight in the simplicity and goodness of cabbage and caraway kraut, a staple ferment that brings a burst of flavor to your culinary creations.

Fermented Jalapeño Peppers

Description: Spice up your palate with fermented jalapeño peppers, a zesty and versatile addition to your culinary repertoire. These fermented peppers add a delightful kick to tacos, sandwiches, or any dish that craves a bold flavor profile.

Preparation Time: 15 minutes

Fermentation Time: 7 to 14 days

Servings: 8

Ingredients:

1 pound of fresh jalapeño peppers

2 cloves of garlic, peeled and sliced

1 tablespoon sea salt

Filtered water

Instructions:

Prepare Jalapeños:

Wash and slice the jalapeños into rounds, or leave them whole for milder heat.

Pack the Jar:

Tightly pack the jalapeño slices into a sterilized jar, interspersing them with sliced garlic.

Create Brine:

In a separate container, dissolve sea salt in filtered water to create a brine solution.

Cover with brine.

Pour the brine over the jalapeños, ensuring they are fully submerged. Leave some headspace in the jar.

Seal the Jar:

Seal the jar with an airtight lid to create an anaerobic environment for fermentation.

Fermentation:

Let the jar ferment at room temperature for 7 to 14 days. Check for the desired level of tanginess and spice.

Taste and refrigerate:

Taste a small portion to determine if the peppers have reached the desired flavor. Refrigerate to slow down fermentation.

Serve and enjoy:

Add fermented jalapeño peppers to tacos, nachos, or any dish that could use a fiery kick.

Tips for beginners:

Gloves for Handling: Wear gloves when handling jalapeños to avoid skin irritation.

Health Benefits:

Probiotic Punch: Fermented jalapeños provide probiotics for gut health.

Vitamin C Boost: Jalapeños are rich in vitamin C, contributing to immune support.

Experience the bold and tangy flavor of fermented jalapeño peppers, a homemade condiment that adds flair to your favorite dishes.

Brussels sprouts and mustard seeds

Description: Elevate the humble Brussels sprouts with the vibrant flavor of mustard seeds in this Fermented Brussels Sprouts recipe. The tangy, crunchy result is a delightful addition to salads, bowls, or enjoyed as a standalone snack.

Preparation Time: 20 minutes

Fermentation Time: 10 to 14 days

Servings: 6

Ingredients:

1 pound of cleaned Brussels sprouts, trimmed and halved

1 tablespoon of mustard seeds

2 cloves of garlic, peeled and minced

1 tablespoon sea salt

Filtered water

Instructions:

Prepare Brussels sprouts:

 Brussels sprouts in half after trimming the ends.

Pack the Jar:

Tightly pack the halved Brussels sprouts into a sterilized jar, interspersing them with mustard seeds and minced garlic.

Create Brine:

In a separate container, dissolve sea salt in filtered water to create a brine solution.

Cover with brine.

Pour the brine over the Brussels sprouts, ensuring they are fully submerged. Leave some headspace in the jar.

Seal the Jar:

Seal the jar with an airtight lid to create an anaerobic environment for fermentation.

Fermentation:

Let the jar ferment at room temperature for 10 to 14 days. Check for the desired level of tanginess and crunch.

Taste and refrigerate:

Taste a small portion to determine if the Brussels sprouts have reached the desired flavor. Refrigerate to slow down fermentation.

Serve and enjoy:

Incorporate fermented Brussels sprouts into salads or grain bowls, or enjoy them as a flavorful snack.

Tips for beginners:

Consistent Sizing: Aim for consistent sizing of Brussels sprouts for even fermentation.

Experiment with Spices: Feel free to experiment with additional spices for a personalized touch.

Health Benefits:

Probiotic Goodness: Fermented Brussels sprouts contribute to a healthy gut with probiotics.

Nutrient-rich: Brussels sprouts are packed with vitamins, fiber, and antioxidants.

Discover the enticing combination of Brussels sprouts and mustard seeds, a fermented treat that transforms a simple vegetable into a flavorful sensation.

CHAPTER 7: FERMENTED CONDIMENT RECIPES

Fermented Tomato Ketchup

Description: Upgrade your condiment game with this fermented tomato ketchup, a tangy and probiotic-rich alternative to store-bought options. Elevate your burgers, fries, and favorite dishes with the robust flavor of naturally fermented tomatoes.

Preparation Time: 20 minutes

Fermentation Time: 7 to 10 days

Servings: 16 (2 tablespoons per serving).

Ingredients:

2 pounds of ripe tomatoes, chopped

1 small onion, finely chopped

2 cloves garlic, minced

1/4 cup raw honey or maple syrup

1/4 cup apple cider vinegar

1 teaspoon sea salt

1/4 teaspoon black pepper

Pinch of cayenne pepper (optional, for heat)

Instructions:

Prepare Tomatoes:

Chop ripe tomatoes, removing seeds if desired.

Create Base:

In a large bowl, combine chopped tomatoes, finely chopped onion, minced garlic, raw honey or maple syrup, apple cider vinegar, sea salt, black pepper, and cayenne pepper if adding.

Blend or Process:

Use an immersion blender or food processor to blend the mixture until smooth.

Pack the Jar:

Transfer the blended mixture into a sterilized jar, leaving some headspace.

Fermentation Lock:

Place a fermentation weight or a clean, small jar filled with water on top of the ketchup to keep it submerged.

Fermentation:

Allow the ketchup to ferment at room temperature for 7 to 10 days. Taste for the desired tanginess.

Strain (Optional):

If a smoother consistency is preferred, strain the ketchup using a fine-mesh strainer.

Refrigerate:

Once fermented, refrigerate the ketchup to slow down the fermentation process.

Serve and enjoy:

Use fermented tomato ketchup as a flavorful condiment for burgers, fries, and various dishes.

Tips for beginners:

Check Daily: Taste the ketchup daily during fermentation to achieve the desired flavor.

Health Benefits:

Probiotic Boost: Fermentation adds probiotics, supporting gut health.

Natural Sweeteners: Raw honey or maple syrup provides sweetness without refined sugars.

Enhance your meals with the wholesome goodness of fermented tomato ketchup, a probiotic-packed condiment that brings a burst of flavor to your favorite dishes.

Tangy fermented mustard

Description: Elevate your culinary creations with this tangy fermented mustard. Packed with bold flavors and the goodness of fermentation, it's a condiment that adds a zesty kick to sandwiches, dressings, and more.

Preparation Time: 15 minutes

Fermentation Time: 5 to 7 days

Servings: 24 (1 tablespoon per serving)

Ingredients:

1 cup of yellow mustard seeds

1/2 cup brown mustard seeds

1 cup apple cider vinegar

1/2 cup of filtered water

1 teaspoon sea salt

1 tablespoon of maple syrup or raw honey.

1/2 teaspoon turmeric powder (optional, for color)

Instructions:

Soak Mustard Seeds:

In a bowl, combine the yellow and brown mustard seeds. Cover with apple cider vinegar and filtered water. Let them soak overnight or at least 8 hours

Blend mustard seeds:

After soaking, blend the mustard seeds with the soaking liquid until you achieve a smooth consistency.

Create Mustard Paste:

Transfer the blended mixture to a bowl and add sea salt, raw honey or maple syrup, and turmeric powder if using. Stir and mix very well to form a thick paste.

Pack the Jar:

Transfer the mustard paste into a sterilized jar, leaving some headspace.

Fermentation Lock:

Place a fermentation weight or a clean, small jar filled with water on top of the mustard paste to keep it submerged.

Fermentation:

Allow the mustard to ferment at room temperature for 5 to 7 days. Taste for the desired tanginess.

Adjust Consistency:

If the mustard is too thick, you can add a little water to achieve the desired consistency.

Refrigerate:

Once fermented, refrigerate the Tangy Fermented Mustard to slow down the fermentation process.

Serve and enjoy:

Use this zesty mustard to enhance the flavor of sandwiches, dressings, or your favorite dishes.

Tips for beginners:

Experiment with Spice: Add a pinch of additional spices like garlic powder or smoked paprika for a personalized touch.

Health Benefits:

Probiotic Punch: Fermented mustard introduces beneficial bacteria for gut health.

Turmeric Boost: Optional turmeric provides a vibrant color and potential anti-inflammatory benefits.

Craft your own tangy fermented mustard at home, infusing your dishes with a burst of flavor and the nutritional benefits of fermentation.

Pickle-Infused Relish

Description: Transform your condiment game with this pickle-infused relish, a delightful blend of sweet and tangy flavors with the crunch of fermented vegetables. Perfect for hot dogs, burgers, and sandwiches, it's a condiment that takes your meals to the next level.

Preparation Time: 20 minutes

Fermentation Time: 5 to 7 days

Servings: 16 (2 tablespoons per serving).

Ingredients:

2 cups finely chopped cucumbers

1/2 cup finely chopped red bell pepper

1/2 cup finely chopped onion

1/4 cup apple cider vinegar

1/4 cup of filtered water

2 table spoonful of maple syrup or raw honey

1 teaspoon of mustard seeds

1/2 teaspoon celery seeds

1/2 teaspoon sea salt

Instructions:

Prepare Vegetables:

Finely chop cucumbers, red bell peppers, and onions.

Create Pickling Liquid:

In a bowl, combine apple cider vinegar, filtered water, raw honey or maple syrup, mustard seeds, celery seeds, and sea salt. Mix well.

Pack the Jar:

Layer the finely chopped vegetables in a sterilized jar, alternating between cucumbers, red bell peppers, and onions.

Pour Pickling Liquid:

Pour the prepared pickling liquid over the vegetables, ensuring they are fully submerged. Leave about 1/2 inch of headspace.

Fermentation Lock:

Place a fermentation weight or a clean, small jar filled with water on top of the vegetables to keep them submerged.

Fermentation:

Allow the relish to ferment at room temperature for 5 to 7 days. Taste for the desired balance of sweetness and tanginess.

Refrigerate:

Once fermented, refrigerate the pickle-infused relish to slow down the fermentation process.

Serve and enjoy:

Use this relish to add a burst of flavor to hot dogs, burgers, sandwiches, or any dish that calls for a zesty relish.

Tips for beginners:

Adjust Sweetness: Taste the relish during fermentation and adjust the sweetness by adding more honey or maple syrup if needed.

Health Benefits:

Fermented Crunch: Enjoy the added crunch and probiotic benefits of fermented vegetables.

Natural Sweeteners: Raw honey or maple syrup provides sweetness without refined sugars.

Craft your own pickle-infused relish at home and experience the joy of a homemade condiment bursting with flavor and the goodness of fermentation.

Homemade fermented Sriracha

Description: Elevate your spice game with this homemade fermented Sriracha. The natural fermentation process enhances the flavor profile, creating a rich and tangy hot sauce that's perfect for adding a kick to your favorite dishes.

Preparation Time: 20 minutes

Fermentation Time: 7 to 10 days

Servings: approximately 16 (1 tablespoon per serving).

Ingredients:

1 pound of red chili peppers, stemmed and halved

4 cloves of garlic, peeled

1 tablespoon light brown sugar

1 tablespoon sea salt

1 cup pineapple, chopped

1/4 cup of filtered water

2 tablespoons fish sauce (optional, for added depth)

1 tablespoon grated ginger

1 tablespoon of rice vinegar

Instructions:

Prepare chili peppers:

Remove the stems from red chili peppers and halve them.

Create a Pepper Mash:

In a blender or food processor, combine red chili peppers, garlic, light brown sugar, and sea salt. Blend the combination until you have a coarse paste.

Initiate Fermentation:

Transfer the pepper mash to a clean, sterilized jar. Press it down to eliminate air pockets.

Prepare the fruit base:

In a separate bowl, combine chopped pineapple, filtered water, fish sauce (if using), grated ginger, and rice vinegar.

Combine and Ferment:

Pour the fruit base over the pepper mash in the jar. Ensure the pepper mash is fully submerged in the liquid.

Fermentation Lock:

Place a fermentation weight or a clean, small jar filled with water on top of the mixture to keep it submerged.

Fermentation Process:

Allow the mixture to ferment at room temperature for 7 to 10 days. Taste for the desired spiciness during the process.

Blend and strain:

After fermentation, blend the mixture until smooth. Strain the liquid using a fine mesh sieve to achieve a smoother Sriracha.

Store and enjoy:

Transfer the strained Sriracha to a clean bottle and refrigerate.

Tips for beginners:

Adjust Spice Level: Taste the Sriracha during fermentation and adjust the spiciness by extending or reducing the fermentation time.

Health Benefits:

Natural Heat: Red chili peppers produce capsaicin, known for its metabolism-boosting and anti-inflammatory properties.

Probiotic Boost: Fermented foods contribute to gut health, supporting digestion and a healthy immune system.

Craft your own homemade fermented Sriracha and savor the unique depth of flavor that fermentation brings to this iconic hot sauce.

Probiotic Salsa Fresca

Description: Give your salsa a probiotic punch with this Probiotic Salsa Fresca. Bursting with fresh ingredients and enhanced by the natural fermentation process, this tangy salsa adds a zesty twist to your favorite snacks and meals.

Preparation Time: 15 minutes

Fermentation Time: 2 to 3 days

Servings: approximately 8 (1/4 cup per serving).

Ingredients:

4 large tomatoes, diced

1 red onion, finely chopped

1 jalapeño pepper, seeded and minced

1/4 cup fresh cilantro, chopped

2 cloves garlic, minced

Juice of 2 limes

1 teaspoon sea salt

1/2 teaspoon black pepper

1/2 teaspoon cumin

1/4 teaspoon cayenne pepper for extra heat(optional)

Instructions:

Prepare fresh ingredients:

Dice the tomatoes, finely chop the red onion, seed and mince the jalapeño pepper, and chop the fresh cilantro.

Combine Ingredients:

In a mixing bowl, combine the diced tomatoes, chopped red onion, minced jalapeño pepper, fresh cilantro, minced garlic, lime juice, sea salt, black pepper, cumin, and cayenne pepper if using.

Mix Thoroughly:

Gently toss the ingredients until well combined, ensuring the flavors meld together.

Transfer to Jar:

Pack the salsa mixture into a clean, sterilized jar, leaving some space at the top.

Press Down:

Press down on the salsa to eliminate air pockets and ensure the liquid covers the ingredients.

Fermentation Lock:

Place a fermentation weight or a small jar filled with water on top to keep the salsa submerged.

Fermentation Process:

Allow the salsa to ferment at room temperature for 2 to 3 days. Taste for the desired tanginess.

Refrigerate and serve:

Once fermented, refrigerate the salsa. Serve chilled and enjoy the probiotic goodness with your favorite dishes.

Tips for beginners:

Adjust Heat: Control the spiciness by adding or omitting cayenne pepper based on your preference.

Health Benefits:

Probiotic Boost: The fermentation process introduces probiotics for improved gut health.

Antioxidant-rich: Tomatoes, onions, and cilantro contribute antioxidants for overall well-being.

Create your own probiotic salsa fresca and experience the vibrant flavors and nutritional benefits of this fermented salsa.

Fermented BBQ Bliss

Description: Elevate your barbecue experience with the tangy kick of Fermented BBQ Bliss. This fermented barbecue sauce brings depth of flavor and probiotic goodness to your grilled favorites, making every bite a savory delight.

Preparation Time: 15 minutes

Fermentation Time: 3 to 5 days

Servings: approximately 12 (2 tablespoons per serving).

Ingredients:

1 cup of ketchup

1/2 cup apple cider vinegar

1/4 cup soy sauce

1/4 cup molasses

1/4 cup brown sugar

2 cloves garlic, minced

1 teaspoon of onion powder

1 teaspoon smoked paprika

1/2 teaspoon cayenne pepper

1/2 teaspoon black pepper

1/4 teaspoon liquid smoke (optional)

Salt to taste

Instructions:

Combine Ingredients:

In a mixing bowl, whisk together ketchup, apple cider vinegar, soy sauce, molasses, brown sugar, minced garlic, onion powder, smoked paprika, cayenne pepper, black pepper, and liquid smoke if using.

Mix Thoroughly:

Ensure all ingredients are well combined, creating a smooth and homogenous mixture.

Transfer to Jar:

Pour the BBQ sauce into a clean, sterilized jar, leaving some space at the top.

Press Down:

Press down on the sauce to eliminate air pockets and ensure it is fully covered with liquid.

Fermentation Lock:

Place a fermentation weight or a small jar filled with water on top to keep the sauce submerged.

Fermentation Process:

Allow the BBQ sauce to ferment at room temperature for 3 to 5 days. Taste for the desired tanginess.

Refrigerate and enjoy:

Once fermented, refrigerate the BBQ sauce. Brush it on grilled meats or use it as a flavorful dipping sauce.

Tips for beginners:

Adjust Sweetness: Fine-tune the sweetness by adding more or less brown sugar according to your taste.

Health Benefits:

Probiotic Infusion: The fermentation process adds probiotics for digestive health.

Flavorful Antioxidants: Garlic, onion, and smoked paprika contribute antioxidant-rich flavors.

Prepare your fermented BBQ sauce to infuse your barbecue gatherings with a burst of flavor and gut-friendly benefits.

Spicy Fermented Hot Sauce

Description: Ignite your taste buds with the fiery kick of Spicy Fermented Hot Sauce. This homemade hot sauce combines the intense heat of peppers with the depth of fermentation, creating a bold condiment to elevate any dish.

Preparation Time: 20 minutes

Fermentation Time: 5 to 7 days

Servings: approximately 16 (1 tablespoon per serving).

Ingredients:

1 cup hot peppers (jalapeños, serranos, or a mix), chopped

1 cup bell peppers (red or orange), chopped

3 cloves garlic, minced

1 small onion, chopped

2 cups of white vinegar

1 tablespoon sea salt

1 teaspoon sugar

Instructions:

Prepare Peppers:

Wear gloves to chop the hot peppers. Remove seeds for milder heat or leave them for extra spiciness.

Combine Ingredients:

In a blender, combine the hot peppers, bell peppers, minced garlic, chopped onion, white vinegar, sea salt, and sugar.

Blend Smooth:

Blend the ingredients until you achieve a smooth consistency.

Transfer to Jar:

Pour the blended mixture into a clean, sterilized jar, leaving some space at the top.

Fermentation Lock:

Cover the jar loosely to allow gasses to escape during fermentation. Use a fermentation weight or small jar filled with water to keep the mixture submerged.

Fermentation Process:

Allow the hot sauce to ferment at room temperature for 5 to 7 days. Taste for the desired spiciness.

Strain and store:

Strain the fermented hot sauce to remove solids. Transfer the liquid to a bottle and store it in the refrigerator.

Enjoy the heat:

Add this spicy, fermented hot sauce to your favorite dishes for an extra kick. Use it sparingly, as it can be intensely hot.

Tips for beginners:

Experiment with pepper varieties to customize the heat level.

Adjust salt and sugar to suit your taste preferences.

Health Benefits:

Probiotic Boost: The fermentation process adds probiotics for gut health.

Antioxidant-rich: Peppers and garlic contribute antioxidants with potential health benefits.

Prepare your spicy fermented hot sauce and turn up the heat on your culinary adventures.

Traditional Miso Elixir

Description: Immerse yourself in the rich umami flavor of Traditional Miso Elixir, a classic fermented concoction with a depth of taste that elevates soups, dressings, and marinades.

Preparation Time: 10 minutes

Fermentation Time: 2 to 3 weeks

Servings: approximately 16 (1 tablespoon per serving).

Ingredients:

1 cup organic soybeans

1 cup rice koji (fermented rice)

1/4 cup sea salt

Instructions:

Prepare Soybeans:

Rinse the soybeans and soak them in water overnight.

Cook Soybeans:

Drain the soaked soybeans and cook them in fresh water until they are soft and easily mashable.

Mash Soybeans:

Mash the cooked soybeans into a paste-like consistency.

Mix with rice koji:

In a large bowl, combine the mashed soybeans with rice koji.

Salt Addition:

Gradually add sea salt while continuing to mix the ingredients thoroughly.

Pack-in Jar:

Pack the mixture into a clean, sterilized jar, leaving some space at the top.

Fermentation Lock:

Cover the jar loosely to allow gasses to escape during fermentation. Use a fermentation weight or small jar filled with water to keep the mixture submerged.

Fermentation Process:

Allow the miso mixture to ferment at room temperature for 2 to 3 weeks. Taste for the desired depth of flavor.

Transfer and store:

Transfer the fermented miso elixir to a sealable container and store it in the refrigerator.

Incorporate in Recipes:

Add a tablespoon of Traditional Miso Elixir to soups, dressings, or marinades for an umami boost.

Tips for beginners:

Ensure a clean and sanitized environment for fermentation.

Experiment with different varieties of soybeans for unique flavor profiles.

Health Benefits:

Probiotic Goodness: Traditional miso is known for its probiotic content, which supports gut health.

Rich in Amino Acids: Soybeans provide essential amino acids, contributing to overall nutritional value.

Unlock the savory essence of Traditional Miso Elixir and infuse your culinary creations with the timeless flavor of fermented miso.

Soy Sauce Symphony

Description: Dive into the complex and savory notes of Soy Sauce Symphony, a fermented masterpiece that adds depth and richness to your dishes. Elevate the umami quotient with this homemade soy sauce.

Preparation Time: 20 minutes

Fermentation Time: 6 months to 1 year

Servings: approximately 24 (1 tablespoon per serving).

Ingredients:

2 cups organic soy sauce (non-GMO)

1/4 cup sea salt

1/4 cup dark brown sugar

1-inch piece of kombu (seaweed)

1 tablespoon of whole black peppercorns

1 tablespoon whole cloves

1 tablespoon crushed coriander seeds

Instructions:

Prepare the soy sauce base:

In a large, clean bowl, combine organic soy sauce, sea salt, and dark brown sugar. Mix properly until the salt and sugar dissolve.

Infuse Flavors:

Add kombu, black peppercorns, cloves, and crushed coriander seeds to the soy sauce mixture. Stir properly to evenly distribute the flavors.

Pack-in Container:

Transfer the soy sauce mixture into a sterilized glass container, ensuring there is some space at the top.

Fermentation Lock:

Cover the container with a tight lid or cloth secured with a rubber band. So gasses can escape during fermentation.

Fermentation Process:

Allow the soy sauce to ferment in a cool, dark place for 6 months to 1 year. Taste periodically for the desired depth of flavor.

Strain and store:

Strain the soy sauce to remove solids and aromatics. Transfer the liquid to a bottle and store it in a cool, dark place.

Incorporate in Recipes:

Use Soy Sauce Symphony in stir-fries, marinades, dipping sauces, and various culinary creations for an authentic umami kick.

Tips for beginners:

Ensure all utensils and containers are thoroughly sanitized to prevent unwanted bacteria.

Health Benefits:

Rich Umami Flavor: Enhance the taste of dishes with the robust umami provided by homemade soy sauce.

Reduced Additives: Homemade soy sauce allows control over ingredients, minimizing unnecessary additives.

Craft your own soy sauce symphony and embark on a flavor journey that transcends the ordinary.

Creamy Fermented Mayonnaise

Description: Elevate your condiment game with Creamy Fermented Mayonnaise, a tangy and probiotic-rich alternative to traditional mayo. Indulge in the smooth texture and delightful flavors that fermentation brings to this kitchen staple.

Preparation Time: 15 minutes

Fermentation Time: 24 hours

Servings: approximately 16 (1 tablespoon per serving).

Ingredients:

1 cup of light olive oil

1 egg, at room temperature

1 tablespoon dijon mustard

1 tablespoon apple cider vinegar

1/2 teaspoon sea salt

1/4 teaspoon sugar (optional for feeding probiotics)

Instructions:

Prepare Ingredients:

Make sure the egg is at room temperature for better emulsification.

Blend egg and mustard:

In a blender or food processor, combine the egg and Dijon mustard. Blend until well mixed.

Slowly add oil.

With the blender on low speed, slowly drizzle in the light olive oil. Continue blending until the mixture thickens.

Add vinegar and salt.

Incorporate apple cider vinegar and sea salt. Run the mixture in a blender until it is smooth and creamy.

Transfer to Jar:

Transfer the mayonnaise to a clean, sterilized jar, leaving some space at the top.

Fermentation Lock:

Cover the jar with a lid or cloth secured with a rubber band . So gasses can escape during fermentation.

Fermentation Process:

Allow the mayonnaise to ferment at room temperature for 24 hours. This step enhances the flavors and introduces probiotics.

Refrigerate:

Once fermented, refrigerate the mayonnaise to halt the fermentation process and preserve the creamy texture.

Incorporate in Recipes:

Enjoy creamy fermented mayonnaise in sandwiches, salads, and as a versatile base for various dressings and sauces.

Tips for beginners:

Use high-quality, light olive oil for a milder flavor.

Adjust salt and sugar according to personal preference.

Health Benefits:

Probiotic Boost: Fermentation introduces beneficial bacteria, promoting gut health.

Natural Ingredients: Homemade mayo allows control over ingredients, avoiding preservatives found in commercial options.

Indulge in the creamy goodness of this probiotic-packed Creamy Fermented Mayonnaise and experience the difference in taste and health benefits.

CHAPTER 8: FERMENTED DRINK AND DAIRY RECIPES

Sparkling citrus kombucha

Description: Quench your thirst with the effervescence of Sparkling Citrus Kombucha, a delightful fermented beverage that combines the tang of kombucha with the refreshing zest of citrus. Enjoy the bubbly goodness while benefiting from the probiotics nurtured during the fermentation process.

Preparation Time: 20 minutes

Fermentation Time: 7–14 days

Servings: Approximately 8 (8-ounce servings)

Ingredients:

4 black tea bags

1 cup granulated sugar

1 SCOBY (Symbiotic Culture of Bacteria and Yeast)

2 cups of starter tea (previously brewed kombucha)

1 cup citrus juice (orange, lemon, or a blend)

Zest of one citrus fruit

Additional citrus slices for garnish (optional)

Instructions:

Prepare sweet tea:

Boil 4 cups of water and steep the black tea bags for 5-7 minutes. Stir in the sugar until dissolved. Allow the tea cool to room temperature.

Combine tea and starter:

In a large glass jar, combine the cooled sweet tea and the starter tea.

Add SCOBY:

Place the scoby on top of the liquid carefully.Ensure your hands are clean to avoid contamination.

Cover and Ferment:

Use a cloth or coffee filter to cover the jar, securing it with a rubber band. Allow the kombucha to ferment at room temperature for 7–14 days. Taste it periodically to achieve your preferred level of tartness.

Prepare Citrus Juice:

Squeeze fresh citrus juice and zest one citrus fruit.

Bottle and Flavor:

Once the kombucha reaches your desired tartness, remove the scoby. Bottle the kombucha, adding citrus juice and zest to each bottle. Leave some space at the top.

Second Fermentation:

Seal the bottles tightly and let them ferment for an additional 3–5 days. This builds carbonation.

Refrigerate:

Refrigerate the kombucha to slow down fermentation. This also enhances the flavor and carbonation.

Serve Chilled:

Serve sparkling citrus kombucha over ice, garnished with citrus slices if desired.

Tips for beginners:

Be patient during fermentation; taste preferences vary, so find your ideal balance.

Experiment with different citrus varieties to discover unique flavor profiles.

Health Benefits:

Probiotic Power: Kombucha is a natural source of probiotics, promoting a healthy gut microbiome.

Vitamin Boost: Citrus adds a dose of vitamin C, known for its immune-boosting properties.

Refresh your senses and nourish your body with the delightful Sparkling Citrus Kombucha—a perfect blend of flavor and wellness.

Fruity Water Kefir Fusion

Description: Dive into a symphony of flavors with Fruity Water Kefir Fusion, a vibrant and effervescent beverage that combines the goodness of water kefir with a burst of fruity delights. This fermented drink not only tingles your taste buds but also brings a plethora of probiotics to support your digestive health.

Preparation Time: 15 minutes

Fermentation Time: 24–48 hours

Servings: Approximately 6 (8-ounce servings)

Ingredients:

1/2 cup water kefir grains

1/2 cup organic cane sugar

4 cups of filtered water

1 cup mixed berries (strawberries, blueberries, raspberries)

1/2 cup chopped mango

1 tablespoon fresh ginger, grated

1 tablespoon dried fruit (apricots, raisins, or figs)

1/4 teaspoon sea salt

Instructions:

Create a sugar solution:

Dissolve the organic cane sugar in filtered water to create a sugar solution. Allow the solution to cool down until it reaches room temperature.

Combine Ingredients:

In a large glass jar, combine the water kefir grains, mixed berries, chopped mango, grated ginger, dried fruit, and sea salt.

Add sugar solution:

Pour the cooled sugar solution into the jar, ensuring all ingredients are well mixed.

Cover and Ferment:

Use a cloth or coffee filter to cover the jars, securing it with a rubber band. Allow the Fruity Water Kefir Fusion to ferment at room temperature for 24–48 hours. Taste it periodically to achieve the desired level of effervescence.

Strain and Bottle:

Strain out the water kefir grains and transfer the liquid into bottles. Leave some space at the top.

Second Fermentation:

Seal the bottles tightly and let them undergo a second fermentation for an additional 24–48 hours. This enhances the fruity flavors and carbonation.

Refrigerate:

Refrigerate the fruity water kefir fusion to slow down fermentation. This also chills and intensifies the fruity notes.

Serve Chilled:

Pour the fruity water kefir over ice and relish the refreshing fusion of flavors.

Tips for beginners:

Experiment with various fruit combinations to discover your favorite fusion.

Adjust the fermentation time to achieve the desired level of carbonation.

Health Benefits:

Gut Wellness: Water kefir contributes to a healthy gut microbiome, supporting digestion.

Antioxidant Boost: Berries and mango infuse the drink with antioxidants, promoting overall well-being.

Quench your thirst and invigorate your senses with Fruity Water Kefir Fusion—a delightful marriage of probiotics and fruity goodness.

Creamy Homemade Yogurt Delight

Description: Indulge in the velvety goodness of Creamy Homemade Yogurt Delight, a luscious treat that brings the satisfaction of crafting your yogurt from scratch. This recipe ensures a smooth and rich texture, offering a perfect canvas for your favorite toppings or enjoying it on its own. Elevate your culinary experience with this delightful and nutritious homemade yogurt.

Preparation Time: 15 minutes

Incubation Time: 6–12 hours

Chilling Time: 4 hours

Servings: approximately 4 cups

Ingredients:

4 cups of whole milk

2 tablespoons plain yogurt with live active cultures (as a starter)

Instructions:

Heat Milk:

Pour the whole milk into a saucepan and heat it over medium heat until it reaches just below boiling, around 200°F (93°C). Stir frequently to prevent scalding.

Cool Milk:

Allow the heated milk cool to around 110°F (43°C). This is an ideal temperature for the yogurt culture to thrive.

Add Starter:

In a small bowl, mix the plain yogurt with a small amount of the cooled milk to create a smooth blend. Add this mixture back into the saucepan with the rest of the cooled milk. Stir thoroughly to distribute the yogurt culture evenly.

Incubate:

Pour the milk and yogurt mixture into a clean, airtight container. Cover it and place it in a warm environment for incubation. This can be achieved in an oven with the light on, a yogurt maker, or an insulated cooler. Allow it to incubate for 6–12 hours, or until the yogurt achieves the desired thickness.

Check Consistency:

Check the yogurt's thickness after the incubation period. If it's not set to your liking, you can let it incubate for an additional time.

Chill:

Transfer the container to the refrigerator and let the yogurt chill for at least 4 hours to enhance its creamy texture.

Serve:

Spoon the creamy homemade yogurt delight into bowls and savor the rich, homemade goodness. Top with your favorite fruits, nuts, or honey for added indulgence.

Tips for beginners:

Use high-quality whole milk for a creamier texture.

Ensure the yogurt starter contains live, active cultures for successful fermentation.

Health Benefits:

Probiotic Boost: Homemade yogurt is a natural source of probiotics, promoting a healthy gut.

Nutrient-Rich: Packed with calcium, protein, and beneficial bacteria, this yogurt delight is a nutritious addition to your diet.

Enjoy the satisfaction of creating your own creamy homemade yogurt delight—a delectable masterpiece that tantalizes your taste buds and nurtures your well-being.

Zesty Fermented Lemonade

Description: Quench your thirst with the invigorating kick of Zesty Fermented Lemonade, a sparkling and probiotic-rich beverage that transforms traditional lemonade into a tangy and effervescent delight. Harness the power of fermentation to elevate your drink, creating a refreshing balance of sweet and sour with a twist of zest. Embrace the zestiness and let your taste buds dance with joy.

Preparation Time: 15 minutes

Fermentation Time: 48 hours

Servings: Approximately 6 (8-ounce servings)

Ingredients:

6 organic lemons, juiced

1/4 cup honey

1/2 teaspoon grated ginger

1/4 teaspoon sea salt

6 cups of filtered water

Instructions:

Prepare lemon juice:

Squeeze the juice from the organic lemons, ensuring to strain out any seeds.

Sweeten the lemonade:

In a large mixing bowl, combine the freshly squeezed lemon juice, granulated sugar, honey, grated ginger, and sea salt. Mix well until the honey is fully dissolved.

Dilute with water:

Gradually add filtered water to the lemonade mixture, stirring continuously. Make sure the tastes are dispersed equally.

Transfer to Jar:

Pour the zesty lemonade into a clean glass jar, leaving some space at the top.

Cover and Ferment:

Seal the jar with a tight-fitting lid. Allow the Zesty Fermented Lemonade to ferment at room temperature for 48 hours. Check the taste periodically to achieve the desired level of tartness and effervescence.

Strain (Optional):

If desired, strain the fermented lemonade to remove any pulp or zest. This is optional, depending on your personal preference.

Refrigerate:

Once the fermentation process is complete, refrigerate the lemonade to slow down fermentation and chill the drink.

Serve Chilled:

Pour the Zesty Fermented Lemonade over ice and relish the zingy and fizzy goodness. Garnish with a slice of lemon for an extra burst of flavor.

Tips for beginners:

Experiment with different honey varieties for unique flavor notes.

Adjust the fermentation time based on your preferred level of fizziness.

Health Benefits:

Probiotic Power: The fermentation process enhances the lemonade with probiotics, promoting gut health.

Immune Boost: Lemons contribute vitamin C, known for its immune-boosting properties.

Delight in the bold flavors of Zesty Fermented Lemonade—a tantalizing fusion of zestiness and effervescence that will leave you refreshed and revitalized.

Ginger Infusion Bliss

Description: Embark on a journey of bold and soothing flavors with Ginger Infusion Bliss, a homemade ginger beer that combines the fiery warmth of ginger with the effervescence of fermentation.

Preparation Time: 20 minutes

Fermentation Time: 3–5 days

Servings: Approximately 8 (8-ounce servings)

Ingredients:

2 cups fresh ginger, peeled and grated

1 cup organic cane sugar

1 cup of fresh lemon juice

1/4 teaspoon cayenne pepper for extra heat (optional)

8 cups of filtered water

1/2 cup ginger beer (or use 1/4 cup whey or a commercial ginger beer culture)

Instructions:

Prepare Ginger Syrup:

In a saucepan, combine the grated ginger, organic cane sugar, and filtered water. Bring to a gentle boil, stirring until the sugar is completely dissolved. Simmer for 10 minutes to infuse the flavors.

Cool Ginger Syrup:

Allow the ginger syrup to cool to room temperature. Strain out the ginger solids, leaving a smooth syrup.

Add lemon juice.

Stir in the fresh lemon juice and cayenne pepper (if using) into the ginger syrup.

Introduce the Ginger Bug:

Add the ginger bug to the ginger-lemon mixture. If you don't have a ginger bug, you can use whey or a commercial ginger beer culture as an alternative.

Mix Thoroughly:

Ensure the ingredients are well combined, creating a homogenous ginger-infused liquid.

Transfer to the Fermentation Container:

Pour the ginger infusion into a clean, airtight fermentation container, leaving some space at the top.

Cover and Ferment:

Seal the container and let it ferment at room temperature for 3–5 days. Check the ginger beer daily and press down any foam that may develop during fermentation.

Strain (Optional):

Strain the ginger beer to remove any residual ginger particles, ensuring a smoother texture. This is optional and depends on preferences.

Bottle and carbonate (optional):

If desired, transfer the ginger beer into bottles, leaving some space at the top. Seal it tightly and let it carbonate for an additional day.

Refrigerate:

Refrigerate the Ginger Infusion Bliss to halt fermentation and enhance the flavors. This also results in a chilled and refreshing beverage.

Serve Chilled:

Pour the ginger beer over ice and relish the spicy-sweet notes of your homemade ginger infusion bliss.

*Note: To make a ginger bug, mix 2 tablespoons grated ginger, 2 tablespoons organic cane sugar, and 2 cups water in a jar. Feed it daily with an additional tablespoon each of ginger and sugar for about a week until bubbly.

Tips for beginners:

Adjust the ginger and sugar quantities to suit your preferred level of spiciness and sweetness.

Experiment with different fermentation times for varying levels of carbonation.

Health Benefits:

Digestive Aid: Ginger is known for its digestive properties, making this ginger beer soothing and beneficial for the stomach.

Immune Support: The combination of ginger and lemon provides a boost to the immune system.

Craft your own Ginger Infusion Bliss and discover the delightful harmony of homemade ginger beer—a fusion of bold flavors that will invigorate your senses and leave you in blissful satisfaction.

Fermented Mango Lassi Elixir

Description: Immerse yourself in the tropical paradise of Naturally Fermented Mango Lassi Elixir, a luxurious and probiotic-rich beverage that seamlessly blends the succulence of ripe mangoes with the velvety richness of yogurt. Indulge in the refreshing taste of this classic Indian-inspired drink that doubles as a soothing treat.

Preparation Time: 10 minutes

Fermentation Time: 24-48 hours

Servings: approximately 4 cups

Ingredients:

2 ripe mangoes, peeled, pitted, and diced

2 cups of plain yogurt

1/4 cup honey (adjust to taste)

1/2 teaspoon ground cardamom

1/2 teaspoon vanilla extract

1 cup of ice cubes (optional)

Mint leaves for garnish (optional)

Instructions:

Prepare Mangoes:

Peel, pit, and dice the ripe mangoes.

Blend Mangoes:

In a blender, combine the diced mangoes, plain yogurt, honey, ground cardamom, and vanilla extract. Blend the combination until it is smooth and creamy.

Fermentation:

Transfer the mango-yogurt mixture into a clean, airtight fermentation container. Allow it to ferment at room temperature for 24–48 hours. This natural fermentation process will introduce probiotics to the elixir.

Adjust Sweetness:

Taste the fermented mango lassi elixir and adjust the sweetness by adding more honey if needed. Blend again to incorporate any adjustments.

Chill:

If desired, refrigerate the elixir for an hour to enhance its chill factor.

Serve:

Pour the Naturally Fermented Mango Lassi Elixir into glasses. Add ice cubes if you like a colder drink.

Garnish (Optional):

Garnish the elixir with mint leaves for a refreshing touch.

Enjoy:

Savor the velvety goodness of Naturally Fermented Mango Lassi Elixir, a perfect blend of mangoes and yogurt, now naturally infused with probiotics.

Tips for beginners:

Ensure your fermentation container is clean and sanitized.

Adjust the fermentation time based on your taste preferences and desired level of probiotic activity.

Health Benefits:

Probiotics: The fermentation process naturally introduces beneficial probiotics, promoting a healthy gut microbiome.

Nutrient-rich: mangoes are packed with vitamins, while yogurt adds protein and additional probiotics.

Immerse yourself in the exotic allure of Naturally Fermented Mango Lassi Elixir—a delightful elixir that combines the richness of mangoes with the smoothness of yogurt and the inherent benefits of natural probiotics.

Dairy-Free Coconut Yogurt Marvel

Description: Embark on a dairy-free journey with Coconut Yogurt Marvel, a creamy and probiotic-rich alternative that captures the tropical essence of coconut. Craft your own velvety yogurt, perfect for those seeking a non-dairy indulgence. Experience the marvel of natural fermentation as coconut milk transforms into a luscious, gut-friendly delight.

Preparation Time: 15 minutes

Fermentation Time: 24-48 hours

Servings: approximately 4 cups

Ingredients:

2 cans (800 ml) of full-fat coconut milk

2 tablespoons of tapioca starch or arrowroot powder

2 tablespoons of maple syrup or agave nectar

Instructions:

Prepare the coconut milk base:

Shake the cans of coconut milk well. In a saucepan, heat one can of coconut milk over medium heat. Dissolve arrowroot powder or tapioca starch in the second can of coconut milk. Once the first can is heated, add the starch-milk mixture and stir until thickened. Allow it to cool down until it reaches room temperature.

Sweeten the mixture:

Stir in maple syrup or agave nectar into the cooled coconut milk mixture. Ensure the sweetness is evenly distributed.

Transfer to the Fermentation Container:

Pour the coconut milk mixture into a clean, airtight fermentation container, leaving some space at the top.

Fermentation:

Seal the container and let it ferment at room temperature for 24–48 hours. Check periodically for the desired thickness and probiotic activity.

Refrigerate:

Once the Coconut Yogurt Marvel reaches your preferred consistency, refrigerate it to slow down fermentation. This also chills and enhances the flavor of the yogurt.

Serve:

Scoop the dairy-free coconut yogurt into bowls. Enjoy it as is, or add your favorite toppings, such as fresh fruit or a drizzle of honey.

Tips for beginners:

Use probiotic capsules with a variety of strains for enhanced probiotic diversity.

Experiment with fermentation times to achieve the desired level of tanginess and thickness.

Health Benefits:

Probiotic Power: Coconut Yogurt Marvel is a natural source of probiotics, supporting a healthy gut microbiome.

Dairy-Free Delight: Perfect for individuals with lactose intolerance or those seeking a plant-based alternative.

Experience the marvel of natural fermentation with Dairy-Free Coconut Yogurt Marvel—a creamy, dairy-free indulgence teeming with gut-friendly probiotics and the tropical allure of coconut.

Tangy Buttermilk Brew

Description: Dive into the tangy sensation of Tangy Buttermilk Brew, a probiotic-rich beverage that combines the refreshing taste of buttermilk with the zing of natural fermentation. Craft your own delightful brew, perfect for sipping on its own or as a versatile ingredient in your culinary endeavors. Experience the natural tanginess and gut-friendly goodness with each sip of this fermented buttermilk marvel.

Preparation Time: 10 minutes

Fermentation Time: 12–24 hours

Servings: approximately 4 cups

Ingredients:

4 cups of whole milk

2 tablespoons plain yogurt with live active cultures (as a starter)

1/2 teaspoon salt

Fresh herbs for garnish (optional)

Instructions:

Heat the milk.

In a saucepan, heat the whole milk over medium heat until it reaches just below boiling, around 200°F (93°C). Stir frequently to prevent scalding.

Cool the milk:

Allow the heated milk cool to around 110°F (43°C). This is an ideal temperature for the buttermilk culture to thrive.

Add Starter:

In a small bowl, mix the plain yogurt with a small amount of the cooled milk to create a smooth blend. Add this mixture back into the saucepan with the rest of the cooled milk. Stir thoroughly to distribute the buttermilk culture evenly.

Salt the mixture:

Stir in the salt, ensuring it is well incorporated into the milk mixture.

Fermentation:

Pour the buttermilk mixture into a clean, airtight fermentation container. Allow it to ferment at room temperature for 12–24 hours, or until it achieves the desired thickness and tanginess.

Check Consistency:

After the fermentation period, check the buttermilk for thickness and tanginess. If it's not set to your liking, you can let it ferment for an additional time.

Refrigerate:

Once the Tangy Buttermilk Brew reaches your preferred consistency, refrigerate it to halt fermentation. This also chills and intensifies the tangy flavor.

Serve:

Pour the tangy buttermilk brew into glasses. Garnish with fresh herbs, if desired.

Tips for beginners:

Use high-quality whole milk for a creamier texture.

Adjust the fermentation time based on your preferred level of tanginess.

Health Benefits:

Probiotic Boost: Tangy Buttermilk Brew is a natural source of probiotics, promoting a healthy gut microbiome.

Calcium and Protein: Buttermilk provides essential nutrients like calcium and protein.

Indulge in the natural tanginess and gut-friendly goodness of Tangy Buttermilk Brew—a refreshing and versatile fermented beverage that elevates your taste buds and supports digestive well-being.

Jasmine Blossom Jun Tea

Description: Immerse yourself in the delicate aroma of Jasmine Blossom Jun Tea, a fragrant and effervescent beverage that marries the ancient traditions of kombucha with the floral notes of jasmine. Craft your own exquisite brew, blending the benefits of green tea, honey, and the artistry of natural fermentation. Sip and savor the floral symphony that unfolds with each sparkling drop of this jasmine-infused jun tea.

Preparation Time: 15 minutes

Fermentation Time: 7–14 days

Servings: Approximately 8 (8-ounce servings)

Ingredients:

4 green tea bags

1 cup of honey

1 SCOBY (Symbiotic Culture of Bacteria and Yeast)

2 cups of jun tea starter (previously brewed jun tea)

1/4 cup jasmine blossoms (dried or fresh)

Zest of one lemon (optional)

Additional jasmine blossoms for garnish (optional)

Instructions:

Prepare green tea:

Boil 4 cups of water and steep the green tea bags for 3–5 minutes. Remove the tea bags and allow the tea to cool down reaching room temperature.

Add Honey:

Stir in the honey until it completely dissolves in the green tea. This sweetened tea will be the base for your Jasmine Blossom Jun Tea.

Infuse with Jasmine:

Add the jasmine blossoms to the sweetened green tea. If using dried blossoms, ensure they are clean and free of debris. Allow the tea to infuse with the jasmine aroma for at least 30 minutes.

Strain and Cool:

Strain out the jasmine blossoms and allow the sweetened, jasmine-infused green tea to cool to room temperature.

Combine with Starter and SCOBY:

In a large glass jar, combine the cooled jasmine-infused green tea with the jun tea starter. Place the spoon on top of the liquid gently.

Cover and Ferment:

Use a cloth or coffee filter to cover the jars, securing them with a rubber band. Allow the Jasmine Blossom Jun Tea to ferment at room temperature for 7–14 days. Taste it periodically to achieve your preferred level of tartness.

Zest of Lemon (Optional):

If desired, add the zest of one lemon to the jun tea during the fermentation process for a citrusy twist.

Bottle and Strain (Optional):

Once the desired tartness is reached, remove the scoby. Bottle the Jasmine Blossom Jun Tea, straining out any remaining jasmine blossoms if preferred.

Second Fermentation:

Seal the bottles tightly and let them ferment for an additional 3–5 days. This builds carbonation.

Refrigerate:

Refrigerate the bottled Jasmine Blossom Jun Tea to slow down fermentation and enhance the flavor and carbonation.

Serve Chilled:

Pour the Jasmine Blossom Jun Tea into glasses, garnish with additional jasmine blossoms if desired, and enjoy the effervescent beauty of this floral-infused brew.

Tips for beginners:

Experiment with the quantity of jasmine blossoms to find your desired level of floral aroma.

Be patient during fermentation; taste preferences vary, so find your ideal balance.

Health Benefits:

Probiotic Power: Jasmine Blossom Jun tea is a natural source of probiotics, promoting a healthy gut microbiome.

Antioxidant Boost: Green tea and jasmine contribute antioxidants, supporting overall well-being.

Indulge in the fragrant and effervescent delight of Jasmine Blossom Jun Tea—a sparkling fusion of floral notes and probiotic richness that will elevate your tea experience.

Cinnamon-Spiced Fermented Horchata

Description: Embark on a flavorful journey with Cinnamon-Spiced Fermented Horchata, a unique twist on the traditional Mexican rice and cinnamon drink. Infused with the warmth of cinnamon and enhanced by the magic of natural fermentation, this fermented horchata offers a probiotic-rich, spiced delight.

Preparation Time: 15 minutes

Fermentation Time: 24-48 hours

Servings: approximately 6 cups

Ingredients:

1 cup long-grain white rice

4 cups of water

1 cinnamon stick

1/2 cup cane sugar (adjust to taste)

1/2 cup unsweetened almond milk (or any non-dairy milk of your choice)

1/2 teaspoon vanilla extract

1/4 teaspoon ground cinnamon (for extra spice)

1/4 cup water kefir grains or 1/4 cup jun tea starter

Instructions:

Prepare the rice mixture:

Rinse the white rice thoroughly. In a blender, combine the rinsed rice, water, and the cinnamon stick. Blend the combination, but not completely smooth.

Infuse with cinnamon:

Pour the rice mixture into a clean container, and add the ground cinnamon. Stir well and allow the mixture to sit at room temperature for 2-4 hours to infuse the cinnamon flavor.

Strain the rice mixture.

Strain the rice mixture using a fine-mesh sieve or cheesecloth, separating the liquid from the rice solids. Throw away the solids or save them for another use.

Sweeten and Flavor:

Add cane sugar, almond milk, and vanilla extract to the strained rice liquid. Stir the mixture very well until the sugar is fully dissolved.

Inoculate with Fermentation Starter:

Add water, kefir grains, or jun tea starter to the sweetened rice liquid. Ensure they are well distributed.

Transfer to the Fermentation Container:

Pour the sweetened and inoculated rice liquid into a clean, airtight fermentation container.

Fermentation:

Seal the container and let it ferment at room temperature for 24–48 hours. Check periodically for the desired level of sweetness and effervescence.

Strain and chill:

Strain out any solids or grains from the fermented horchata. Refrigerate the liquid to halt fermentation and chill the drink.

Serve over ice:

Pour the cinnamon-spiced fermented horchata over ice. Sprinkle a dash of ground cinnamon on top for an extra layer of spice.

Tips for beginners:

Adjust the sugar quantity to suit your sweetness preference.

Experiment with the fermentation time for varying levels of effervescence.

Health Benefits:

Probiotic Enrichment: Cinnamon-Spiced Fermented Horchata is a natural source of probiotics, contributing to a healthy gut microbiome.

Dairy-Free Delight: Perfect for those seeking a non-dairy, probiotic-rich alternative.

Savor the delightful combination of cinnamon-spiced warmth and natural fermentation with Cinnamon-Spiced Fermented Horchata—a probiotic-rich take on a classic Mexican beverage.

CHAPTER 9 : FERMENTED FRUIT RECIPES

Fermented Berry Medley

Description: Immerse your taste buds in a vibrant burst of flavors with Fermented Berry Medley, a delightful fusion of assorted berries elevated by the magic of natural fermentation. Packed with antioxidants and probiotics, this fermented fruit medley is a healthy and refreshing addition to your culinary repertoire.

Preparation Time: 15 minutes

Fermentation Time: 3–5 days

Servings: approximately 4 cups

Ingredients:

2 cups mixed berries (strawberries, blueberries, raspberries, and blackberries)

1 tablespoon of honey or maple syrup

1/2 teaspoon sea salt

1/4 teaspoon grated ginger

1/4 teaspoon cinnamon (optional)

1/4 cup water kefir or whey (from strained yogurt)

Instructions:

Prepare Berries:

Rinse the mixed berries thoroughly, and chop the larger berries into bite-sized pieces.

Create Sweetened Brine:

In a bowl, combine honey or maple syrup, sea salt, grated ginger, and cinnamon (if using). Mix well to create a sweetened brine.

Coat Berries:

Toss the mixed berries in the sweetened brine, ensuring they are well coated. Let them sit for 10 minutes to allow the berries to release some juice.

Transfer to the Fermentation Container:

Place the coated berries along with any released juice into a clean, airtight fermentation container.

Inoculate with Probiotics:

Add water, kefir, or whey to the berries. Ensure even distribution for consistent fermentation.

Seal and Ferment:

Seal the fermentation container and let the berries ferment at room temperature for 3–5 days. Stir the mixture daily to prevent the growth of mold and ensure even fermentation.

Taste Check:

After 3 days, taste the fermented berry medley. If it has reached your desired level of sweetness and tanginess, it's ready. If not, continue fermenting for an additional day or two.

Refrigerate:

Once fermented to your liking, refrigerate the Fermented Berry Medley to halt fermentation. This also enhances the flavor and prolongs the shelf life.

Serve and enjoy.

Spoon the Fermented Berry Medley over yogurt, blend into smoothies, or enjoy it on its own as a tangy and probiotic-rich fruit medley.

Tips for beginners:

Experiment with different berry combinations to explore unique flavor profiles.

Adjust the fermentation time based on your preferred level of sweetness and tanginess.

Health Benefits:

Antioxidant Boost: The mixed berries provide a variety of antioxidants that contribute to overall well-being.

Probiotic Power: Water kefir or whey adds beneficial probiotics, supporting a healthy gut microbiome.

Dive into the delightful world of Fermented Berry Medley—a burst of fruity goodness enriched by the magic of fermentation, perfect for elevating your breakfasts, snacks, or desserts.

Pineapple Ginger Chutney

Description: Elevate your palate with the zesty and tropical Pineapple Ginger Chutney—a fermented delight that marries the sweetness of pineapple with the warmth of ginger. This vibrant chutney adds a burst of flavor to your meals and introduces the benefits of natural fermentation to your culinary creations.

Preparation Time: 20 minutes

Fermentation Time: 5–7 days

Servings: approximately 2 cups

Ingredients:

2 cups fresh pineapple, diced

1 tablespoon fresh ginger, grated

1 tablespoon of honey or maple syrup

1/2 teaspoon sea salt

1/4 teaspoon cayenne pepper (optional for heat)

1/4 cup pineapple juice (freshly squeezed)

1/4 cup whey (from strained yogurt) or water kefir

Instructions:

Prepare pineapple and ginger:

Peel and dice fresh pineapple. Grate fresh ginger.

Create Sweetened Brine:

In a bowl, combine honey or maple syrup, sea salt, cayenne pepper (if using), and pineapple juice. Mix well to create a sweetened brine.

Mix pineapple and ginger:

Toss the diced pineapple and grated ginger in the sweetened brine, ensuring an even coating.

Transfer to the Fermentation Container:

Place the coated pineapple and ginger into a clean, airtight fermentation container.

Inoculate with Probiotics:

Add whey or water kefir to the pineapple and ginger mixture. Ensure even distribution for consistent fermentation.

Seal and Ferment:

Seal the fermentation container and let the pineapple ginger chutney ferment at room temperature for 5–7 days. Stir the mixture daily to prevent the growth of mold and ensure even fermentation.

Taste Check:

After 5 days, taste the chutney. If it has reached your desired level of sweetness and tanginess, it's ready. If not, continue fermenting for an additional day or two.

Refrigerate:

Once fermented to your liking, refrigerate the pineapple ginger chutney to halt fermentation. This also enhances the flavor and prolongs the shelf life.

Serve and enjoy:

Pair the pineapple ginger chutney with grilled meats and curries, or use it as a topping for appetizers. The zesty flavor and probiotic richness make it a versatile addition to your meals.

Tips for beginners:

Adjust the sweetness and spice levels according to how you like it.

Experiment with using the chutney as a glaze or marinade for meats.

Health Benefits:

Digestive Support: The probiotics from whey or water kefir contribute to a healthy gut microbiome.

Anti-Inflammatory Properties: Ginger is known for its anti-inflammatory and immune-boosting properties.

Experience the vibrant fusion of flavors with Pineapple Ginger Chutney—a fermented condiment that transforms your dishes into a culinary symphony.

Fermented Apple Chutney

Description: Embrace the essence of autumn with Fermented Apple Chutney—a delightful blend of apples, spices, and the nuanced depth of fermentation. This probiotic-rich chutney adds a tangy twist to your dishes, making it a versatile condiment that complements both sweet and savory culinary creations.

Preparation Time: 20 minutes

Fermentation Time: 5–7 days

Servings: approximately 2 cups

Ingredients:

3 cups apples, peeled, cored, and diced

1/2 cup raisins

1/4 cup red onion, finely chopped

1/4 cup honey or maple syrup

1 teaspoon fresh ginger, grated

1/2 teaspoon ground cinnamon

1/4 teaspoon ground cloves

1/4 teaspoon sea salt

1/4 cup apple cider vinegar

1/4 cup whey (from strained yogurt) or water kefir

Instructions:

Prepare Apples:

Peel, core, and dice the apples. Ensure a uniform size for even fermentation.

Combine Ingredients:

In a bowl, combine diced apples, raisins, finely chopped red onion, honey or maple syrup, grated ginger, ground cinnamon, ground cloves, and sea salt. Mix properly to create a flavorful mixture.

Add vinegar and probiotics.

Pour apple cider vinegar over the mixture and add whey or water kefir. Ensure even distribution to introduce probiotics for fermentation.

Transfer to the Fermentation Container:

Place the apple mixture into a clean, airtight fermentation container.

Seal and Ferment:

Seal the fermentation container and let the apple chutney ferment at room temperature for 5–7 days. Stir the mixture daily to prevent mold growth and ensure even fermentation.

Taste Check:

After 5 days, taste the chutney. If it has reached your desired level of sweetness and tanginess, it's ready. If not, continue fermenting for an additional day or two.

Refrigerate:

Once fermented to your liking, refrigerate the fermented apple chutney to halt fermentation. This also enhances the flavor and prolongs the shelf life.

Serve and enjoy:

Pair the fermented apple chutney with cheese or roasted meats, or use it as a delightful topping for crackers. The probiotic kick and complex flavors make it a versatile and delicious addition to your meals.

Tips for beginners:

Adjust the sweetness and spice levels to exactly how you like it.

Experiment with using the chutney as a glaze or side dish for various dishes.

Health Benefits:

Probiotic Power: Fermented Apple Chutney is a natural source of probiotics, contributing to a healthy gut microbiome.

Antioxidant Rich: Apples and spices provide antioxidants, supporting overall well-being.

Embrace the autumn harvest with Fermented Apple Chutney—a probiotic-packed condiment that transforms ordinary dishes into extraordinary culinary delights.

Fermented Mango Salsa

Description: Add a tropical twist to your dishes with Fermented Mango Salsa—a vibrant combination of sweet mangoes, zesty lime, and the probiotic magic of fermentation. This salsa is not only a burst of flavor but also a healthful addition to your meals, infusing them with the benefits of natural fermentation.

Preparation Time: 15 minutes

Fermentation Time: 3–5 days

Servings: approximately 2 cups

Ingredients:

2 ripe mangoes, peeled, pitted, and diced

1/2 cup red onion, finely chopped

1/4 cup fresh cilantro, chopped

1 jalapeño pepper, seeds removed, and finely sliced

Juice of 2 limes

1/2 teaspoon sea salt

1/4 teaspoon cumin powder

1/4 cup water kefir or whey (from strained yogurt)

Instructions:

Prepare mango and vegetables.

Peel, pit, and dice the ripe mangoes. Finely chop the red onion, cilantro, and jalapeño pepper.

Combine Ingredients:

In a bowl, combine diced mangoes, chopped red onion, cilantro, jalapeño pepper, lime juice, sea salt, and cumin powder. Mix well to create a flavorful mango salsa mixture.

Inoculate with Probiotics:

Add water, kefir, or whey to the mango salsa mixture. Ensure even distribution to introduce probiotics for fermentation.

Transfer to the Fermentation Container:

Place the mango salsa mixture into a clean, airtight fermentation container.

Seal and Ferment:

Seal the fermentation container and let the mango salsa ferment at room temperature for 3–5 days. Stir the mixture daily to prevent mold growth and ensure even fermentation.

Taste Check:

After 3 days, taste the salsa. If it has reached your desired level of sweetness and tanginess, it's ready. If not, continue fermenting for an additional day or two.

Refrigerate:

Once fermented to your liking, refrigerate the fermented mango salsa to halt fermentation. This also enhances the flavor and prolongs the shelf life.

Serve and enjoy.

Pair the fermented mango salsa with grilled meats or fish tacos, or enjoy it with tortilla chips. The probiotic kick and tropical flavors make it a versatile and delicious addition to your meals.

Tips for beginners:

Adjust the spiciness and acidity according to your taste preferences.

Experiment with using the salsa as a topping for various dishes.

Health Benefits:

Probiotic Power: Fermented Mango Salsa is a natural source of probiotics, promoting a healthy gut microbiome.

Vitamin Boost: Mangoes and limes contribute vitamins and antioxidants, supporting overall well-being.

Savor the tropical goodness of Fermented Mango Salsa—a probiotic-rich delight that brings a burst of flavor to your table and contributes to your well-being.

Fermented Grapes with Herbs

Description: Elevate the elegance of grapes with the aromatic infusion of herbs in Fermented Grapes with Herbs—a sophisticated and probiotic-rich treat that combines the natural sweetness of grapes with the depth of fermentation. Enjoy these tangy, herb-infused grapes as a delightful snack or as an accompaniment to cheese platters.

Preparation Time: 15 minutes

Fermentation Time: 5–7 days

Servings: approximately 2 cups

Ingredients:

2 cups seedless grapes (red or green)

1 tablespoon fresh rosemary, finely chopped

1 tablespoon of fresh thyme leaves

1/2 teaspoon black peppercorns

1/4 teaspoon sea salt

1/4 teaspoon sugar

1/4 cup water kefir or whey (from strained yogurt)

Instructions:

Prepare Grapes:

Rinse the seedless grapes thoroughly and pat them dry.

Create a herb mixture:

In a bowl, combine finely chopped fresh rosemary, thyme leaves, black peppercorns, sea salt, and sugar. Mix well to create a fragrant herb mixture.

Coat Grapes:

Toss the rinsed and dried grapes in the herb mixture, ensuring they are evenly coated.

Inoculate with Probiotics:

Add water, kefir, or whey to the herb-coated grapes. Ensure even distribution to introduce probiotics for fermentation.

Transfer to the Fermentation Container:

Place the herb-coated grapes into a clean, airtight fermentation container.

Seal and Ferment:

Seal the fermentation container and let the grapes with herbs ferment at room temperature for 5–7 days. Stir the mixture daily to prevent mold growth and ensure even fermentation.

Taste Check:

After 5 days, taste the grapes. If they have reached your desired level of sweetness and tanginess, they're ready. If not, continue fermenting for an additional day or two.

Refrigerate:

Once fermented to your liking, refrigerate the fermented grapes with herbs to halt fermentation. This also enhances the flavor and prolongs the shelf life.

Serve and enjoy:

Enjoy the Fermented Grapes with Herbs as a refreshing and probiotic-rich snack, or elevate your cheese platters with these sophisticated, herb-infused grapes.

Tips for beginners:

Experiment with different herb combinations to explore unique flavor profiles.

Adjust the fermentation time based on your preferred level of sweetness and tanginess.

Health Benefits:

Probiotic Power: Fermented grapes with herbs are a natural source of probiotics, promoting a healthy gut microbiome.

Antioxidant Rich: Grapes and herbs contribute antioxidants, supporting overall well-being.

Experience the refined harmony of flavors with Fermented Grapes with Herbs—a delightful fusion of sweetness, tanginess, and herbal sophistication that adds a touch of elegance to your snacking or entertaining moments.

CHAPTER 10: CREATIVE COMBINATIONS AND ADVANCED TECHNIQUES

10.1 Experimenting with Flavors

Dive into the world of creative fermentation where you can explore the art of experimenting with flavors to elevate your pickling and fermenting journey. Unleash your culinary imagination and delve into advanced techniques and unique combinations that will tantalize your taste buds and make your fermented creations truly exceptional.

Flavor Pairing Basics

Before delving into advanced techniques, let's revisit the basics of flavor pairing. Understanding the interplay of sweet, salty, sour, bitter, and umami flavors can guide your experimentation. Consider the following when crafting your fermented delights:

Contrast and Complement: Experiment with contrasting and complementary flavors to achieve balance and complexity.

Herb and Spice Infusions: Elevate your creations with herb and spice infusions. From the warmth of cinnamon to the freshness of mint, the possibilities are endless.

Citrus Zest and Juices: Citrus adds a zingy brightness. Experiment with different citrus varieties and their zests to discover unique flavor profiles.

Unique Ingredient Combinations

Now, let's explore some unique ingredient combinations that can spark your creativity:

Savory Herb Fusion: Combine rosemary, thyme, and sage for a savory herb fusion that pairs well with vegetables and pickled delights.

Spiced Fruits: Infuse fruits like peaches or plums with warming spices such as cardamom and cloves for a delightful spiced twist.

Floral Elegance: Introduce floral notes with lavender, chamomile, or elderflower for an elegant and aromatic touch.

Smoky Infusions: Experiment with smoky flavors by adding ingredients like smoked paprika or chipotle peppers for a bold and distinctive profile.

Tea-Infused Ferments: Explore the complexity of fermented teas like oolong or jasmine to create layered and nuanced flavors in your kombuchas and jun teas.

Advanced Techniques

As you venture into advanced techniques, consider the following:

Multi-Stage Fermentation: Combine different stages of fermentation to develop complex flavors. For example, ferment a base ingredient first, then introduce additional elements for a second fermentation.

Barrel-Aged Ferments: Embrace the tradition of barrel aging. Use wooden barrels for fermentation to impart unique flavors and characteristics to your creations.

Wild Fermentation: Allow naturally occurring wild yeasts and bacteria to contribute to your fermentation. This can lead to unpredictable, yet exciting, flavor profiles.

Temperature Control: Experiment with controlling fermentation temperatures to influence the speed and depth of flavor development.

Extended Aging: Let certain ferments age for extended periods to deepen flavors. This is particularly effective with fermented hot sauces, kimchi, and pickles.

Record-Keeping and Documentation

Finally, in the realm of experimentation, meticulous record-keeping is essential. Maintain a fermentation journal, noting ingredient quantities, fermentation times, and flavor profiles. This will serve as a valuable reference for refining your techniques and achieving consistently exceptional results.

10.2 Advanced Fermentation Methods

In this section, explain advanced fermentation methods that go beyond the basics, offering an understanding of the science and artistry of fermentation. These techniques allow you to push the boundaries of flavor development and create truly unique and extraordinary fermented delights.

Controlled Atmospheric Fermentation

Overview:

Controlled atmospheric fermentation involves manipulating the environment in which your fermentations take place. This can include adjusting factors such as temperature, humidity, and gas composition to influence the fermentation process and final flavor profiles.

Application:

Experiment with controlled atmospheric fermentation for precision in flavor development. For instance, controlling the oxygen levels during certain stages of fermentation can lead to nuanced and distinctive results. This method is particularly effective for delicate ferments like fruits, where subtle flavor notes are crucial.

Sequential Fermentation

Overview:

Sequential fermentation is a multi-stage fermentation process where different ingredients or components are introduced at distinct stages. This method allows for the layering of flavors, creating a complex and harmonious end product.

Application:

Consider sequential fermentation for recipes with multiple components. For example, ferment a base ingredient first and then introduce additional elements, such as spices or fruits, for a second fermentation stage. This technique is excellent for achieving depth and complexity in beverages like kombucha or jun tea.

Enzyme-Assisted Fermentation

Overview:

Enzyme-assisted fermentation involves the addition of specific enzymes to enhance the breakdown of complex compounds into simpler, more flavorful components. This method accelerates the fermentation process and can lead to unique taste profiles.

Application:

Experiment with adding natural enzymes like amylase or protease to your ferments. This is particularly effective for breaking down starches into sugars or proteins into amino acids, intensifying the umami and sweetness in your creations.

Hybrid Fermentation

Overview:

Hybrid fermentation combines different fermentation methods within a single recipe. This could involve incorporating both wild fermentation and controlled fermentation processes to achieve a balance between unpredictability and precision.

Application:

Explore the creative possibilities of hybrid fermentation by introducing wild yeasts for the initial stages of fermentation, followed by a controlled fermentation process to refine and shape the final product. This technique is versatile and can be applied to various fermented foods and beverages.

Infusion and Aging in Wood Barrels

Overview:

Infusion and Aging in Wood Barrels introduce the complexities of wood into your ferments. The porous nature of wood allows for a slow and nuanced exchange of flavors between the ferment and the barrel, resulting in a refined end product.

Application:

Select specific types of wood barrels, such as oak or cherry, to impart distinct characteristics to your ferments. This method is commonly used in brewing, winemaking, and vinegar production, contributing to the depth and sophistication of the final product.

Cryo-Fermentation

Overview:

Cryo-fermentation involves freezing the ingredients before fermentation. Freezing ruptures cell walls, allowing for enhanced extraction of flavors and sugars during fermentation.

Application:

Experiment with cryo-fermentation for fruits, herbs, or even vegetables. The freezing process can intensify the natural sugars, resulting in a concentrated and rich flavor profile. This technique is particularly effective for creating complex fruit wines or potent infusions.

Nitro-Fermentation

Overview:

Nitro-fermentation introduces nitrogen gas into the fermentation process. This can influence the texture, effervescence, and overall mouthfeel of the final product.

Application:

Explore nitro-fermentation in beverages like kombucha or beer. The nitrogen infusion creates a velvety texture and enhances the creaminess of the liquid. This method is commonly used in the craft beverage industry to elevate the drinking experience.

As you embark on the journey of advanced fermentation methods, keep in mind that experimentation and observation are key. Document your processes, take notes on flavors and aromas, and allow your creativity to flourish. These advanced techniques open doors to a world of possibilities, allowing you to craft fermented masterpieces that are truly one-of-a-kind.

Conclusion

As we come to the end of our pickling and fermenting journey, let's take a moment to savor the accomplishments and embrace the endless possibilities that lie ahead. Throughout this cookbook, we've embarked on a flavorful expedition, transforming simple ingredients into extraordinary creations through the magic of fermentation. From the bubbling goodness of Sparkling Citrus Kombucha to the savory crunch of Fermented Pickle Relish, each recipe has offered a taste of the diverse and delicious world of fermented foods.

In Chapter 10, we explored advanced techniques, inviting you to become a fermentation maestro in your own kitchen. These methods allow for even more creativity and experimentation, providing a platform for you to put your unique spin on traditional recipes. Whether it's controlled atmospheric fermentation, sequential fermentation, or infusing flavors through wood barrels, the possibilities are as vast as your imagination.

The beauty of pickling and fermenting lies not only in the rich flavors but also in the health benefits these foods bring to our tables. The probiotics cultivated during the fermentation process contribute to a thriving gut microbiome, supporting digestion and overall well-being. Incorporating these probiotic-rich delights into your daily meals is not just a culinary choice; it's a step toward a healthier lifestyle.

As we round off, let's talk about the practical side of things: storing and preserving your fermented treasures. Your homemade creations are a testament to your culinary skills and dedication. Proper storage ensures that the flavors mature gracefully and that you can enjoy the fruits of your labor over an extended period of time.

Now, let's talk about encouragement. The journey of pickling and fermenting is not just about the recipes; it's about the experience and the joy that comes with it. It's about that sense of accomplishment when you taste the first batch of your homemade kimchi or share your homemade kombucha with friends. It's about the thrill of trying something new and the satisfaction of creating food that not only tastes good but is also good for you.

So, to all the home cooks and aspiring fermenters out there, let this be an encouragement to keep going. Don't be afraid to try new recipes, experiment with flavors, and maybe even create your own signature ferments. The world of pickling and fermenting is vast, and your kitchen is your laboratory.

Remember, it's okay if things don't turn out perfect the first time. The beauty of this journey is in the learning process. Each batch teaches you something new about flavors, textures, and the fascinating world of microbes. Celebrate the successes, learn from the mishaps, and, most importantly, enjoy the process.

In the end, it's about the joy of creating something with your hands and the satisfaction of nourishing yourself and your loved ones with wholesome, homemade food. So, here's to your pickling and fermenting journey—may it be filled with delicious discoveries, healthful benefits, and the simple joy of creating something wonderful in your own kitchen. Cheers to the next batch, the next experiment, and the next chapter in your flavorful adventure!